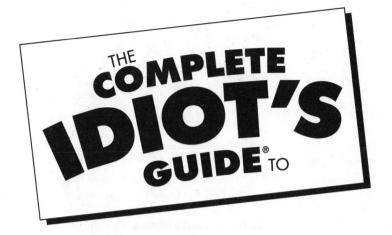

THE COMPLETE IDIOT'S GUIDE® TO

Massage

Illustrated

by Victoria Jordan Stone, CMT, and Bob Shell

ALPHA

A member of Penguin Group (USA) Inc.

ALPHA BOOKS

Published by the Penguin Group

Penguin Group (USA) Inc., 375 Hudson Street, New York, New York 10014, U.S.A.

Penguin Group (Canada), 10 Alcorn Avenue, Toronto, Ontario, Canada M4V 3B2 (a division of Pearson Penguin Canada Inc.)

Penguin Books Ltd, 80 Strand, London WC2R 0RL, England

Penguin Ireland, 25 St Stephen's Green, Dublin 2, Ireland (a division of Penguin Books Ltd)

Penguin Group (Australia), 250 Camberwell Road, Camberwell, Victoria 3124, Australia (a division of Pearson Australia Group Pty Ltd)

Penguin Books India Pvt Ltd, 11 Community Centre, Panchsheel Park, New Delhi—10 017, India

Penguin Group (NZ), cnr Airborne and Rosedale Roads, Albany, Auckland 1310, New Zealand (a division of Pearson New Zealand Ltd)

Penguin Books (South Africa) (Pty) Ltd, 24 Sturdee Avenue, Rosebank, Johannesburg 2196, South Africa

Penguin Books Ltd, Registered Offices: 80 Strand, London WC2R 0RL, England

International Standard Book Number: 978-1-59257-587-9
Library of Congress Catalog Card Number: 2006936694

09 08 07   8 7 6 5 4 3 2 1

Interpretation of the printing code: The rightmost number of the first series of numbers is the year of the book's printing; the rightmost number of the second series of numbers is the number of the book's printing. For example, a printing code of 07-1 shows that the first printing occurred in 2007.

Printed in the United States of America

Note: This publication contains the opinions and ideas of its authors. It is intended to provide helpful and informative material on the subject matter covered. It is sold with the understanding that the authors and publisher are not engaged in rendering professional services in the book. If the reader requires personal assistance or advice, a competent professional should be consulted.

The authors and publisher specifically disclaim any responsibility for any liability, loss, or risk, personal or otherwise, which is incurred as a consequence, directly or indirectly, of the use and application of any of the contents of this book.

Most Alpha books are available at special quantity discounts for bulk purchases for sales promotions, premiums, fund-raising, or educational use. Special books, or book excerpts, can also be created to fit specific needs.

For details, write: Special Markets, Alpha Books, 375 Hudson Street, New York, NY 10014.

Publisher: *Marie Butler-Knight*	**Cartoonist:** *Shannon Wheeler*
Editorial Director: *Mike Sanders*	**Cover Designer:** *Becky Harmon*
Managing Editor: *Billy Fields*	**Book Designers:** *Trina Wurst*
Senior Acquisitions Editor: *Paul Dinas*	**Indexer:** *Julie Bess*
Production Editor: *Megan Douglass*	**Layout:** *Chad Dressler and Becky Harmon*
Copy Editor: *Jan Zoya*	**Proofreader:** *Mary Hunt*

Contents at a Glance

Contents

Introduction

We're living in a high-tech, low-touch society, and as a result, many stressed-out people are touch-deprived, whether they're fully aware of it or not. Massage is a perfect solution, whether performed by a professional or at home between friends and family members. Research has shown tremendous health benefits from massage on all the body's systems for people of all ages.

By following the directions in this book, you'll find that you're able to have the wonderful experience of really helping another person relax, and possibly helping her reduce discomfort she may feel from day-to-day strains, sedentary lifestyle, or energy-intensive activities. Anyone can give massage. Once you know some pretty simple techniques, all you have to do is apply them with warm-hearted intention to help. The receiver will feel warm and cared for, relaxed and glowing, and you'll get to feel good about how you have contributed to their comfort, healing, and ease.

Nobody really knows when the first massage was given. We know that something very like modern massage was performed in ancient Egypt, because tomb art shows beautiful depictions of it. The English word *massage* is derived from the Arabic word *mass'h*, which means "to press gently." Massage has been practiced for thousands of years in China. *The Yellow Emperor's Classic of Internal Medicine*, written in 2700 B.C.E., recommends "massage of skin and flesh" to treat a number of ailments. It's said that Julius Caesar was given a daily massage. In the fifth century B.C.E., Hippocrates, the father of modern medicine, wrote, "The physician must have a wide variety of experience in many things, but particularly in massage, because rubbing can firm a joint that is too loose, and loosen a joint that is too stiff." And Homer wrote about using an oily medium such as olive oil and other salves or ointments for massage. In more recent times, a wide variety of physicians and others mentioned the use of massage in healing practices. Modern massage is usually traced back to Per Heinrich Ling, a fencing master who cured his own arthritis through an organized system of massage and movement, which he called medical gymnastics.

Today, in spite of a proliferation of forms of massage, which have increased exponentially since 1980, the Swedish massage developed from Per Ling's system is still widely practiced. It remains the basic Western massage form to which other therapeutic techniques are added. It's the basic massage method used in most spas today and what we instruct you in here.

In creating this book, our emphasis has been on simplicity wherever possible. We've tried to keep technical terms to an absolute minimum, and we've defined those we felt obliged to use for precision.

After reading this book, watching the DVD, and practicing with friends or family members, you will have skill and confidence to help them with their stress and discomforts. You'll contribute to their health and well-being, as well as your own, because we can't help others without helping ourselves, too. You'll be able to help them relax and enjoy one of the truly finest things in life. Enjoy.

How to Use This Book

We've divided this book into four parts:

To get the most out of this book, you'll need to spend sufficient time in **Part 1, "Massage Basics."** Here we introduce you to massage terminology and the basic massage strokes. Remember to work at a leisurely pace, as there is no profit in rushing through a massage. By taking the time to learn the strokes, you'll ensure that your massages are pleasurable experiences, for both you and the receiver.

When you've learned the strokes, you're ready to move on to a full massage sequence. You'll learn how to combine strokes and work on each area of the body in **Part 2, "Combining Strokes."**

Maybe your intended receiver has a specific problem that can be helped by massage, such as muscle cramps, aching feet, or a sore back. In **Part 3, "Massage Combinations for Specific Problems,"** we teach you techniques to deal with some of these and other common problems.

And finally, in **Part 4, "Taking It Further,"** we give those of you who might want to learn a lot more about massage a good place to start. We hope many of you will like the massage experience so much that you pursue advanced study and professional practice.

We've added two appendixes to the book with sources of supplies and additional information. You should be able to find anything you need there.

How to Use the DVD

Because it's sometimes difficult to visualize the strokes from written description and still photographs, we have provided a DVD with this book. The DVD acquaints you with the main tools we use in these pages. It then takes you through all the strokes so you can clearly see each one and how to properly perform it. Then we have included a condensed version of a full massage you can use as a basis for your own massages. We've also included brief sections on using a mat on the floor instead of a massage table, sitting massage on the floor, massage on a chair, and standing massage. We recommend that you watch the entire DVD a few times to become familiar with it all and then refer to its sections periodically as you learn to perform great massages.

Extras

Throughout this book you'll see asides to the text, especially some cautions and concerns we want to draw your attention to. Here's what to look for:

At Your Fingertips

These sidebars offer tips to help you give a better massage and enhance your massage technique.

Definition

These sidebars define important terms as they are introduced in the text.

Press Here

Massage is not a static art and is constantly changing. These boxes feature the latest information from the world of massage.

Back Off

These warning notes are intended to help you avoid problems and steer clear of situations in which massage is simply not appropriate or must be done with special care. Please read and heed these sidebars.

Acknowledgments

We owe a great debt of thanks to many people who made this book possible. First and foremost we would like to thank Matt Nasta, Certified Rolfer, and Sasha Harrison, Certified Massage Therapist (CMT), our two models; and Natalie Ivanoff, a student at Blue Ridge School of Massage and Yoga, who filled in for some shots when Sasha was not available. Our models worked beyond the call of duty to help us get the best possible images for this book and DVD. The massage tools we feature in Chapter 19 were supplied by Momentum98 (www.momentum98.com), and we really appreciate their help.

Special thanks go to Custom Craftworks (www.customcraftworks.com), makers of the finest massage tables, for supplying the massage table used throughout this book and on the accompanying DVD. Also thanks to Bob Grubel (www.bgrubel.com), who composed and performed the wonderful music we used on the DVD. And a special thank you to Beau Hooker, who was of great help during the photo and video shoots.

Victoria would like to thank Jeff Tiebout, CMT, her original massage instructor, for starting her out on the path of massage, and Faustine Settle, CMT, who mentored her in teaching methods for massage therapy, as well as her fellow instructors, who have shared their teaching methods and massage techniques. She would like to thank the several hundred massage therapy students she has taught over the past 10 years for their input in teaching her how to instruct individuals with all sorts of learning styles and abilities.

Trademarks

All terms mentioned in this book that are known to be or are suspected of being trademarks or service marks have been appropriately capitalized. Alpha Books and Penguin Group (USA) Inc. cannot attest to the accuracy of this information. Use of a term in this book should not be regarded as affecting the validity of any trademark or service mark.

In This Part

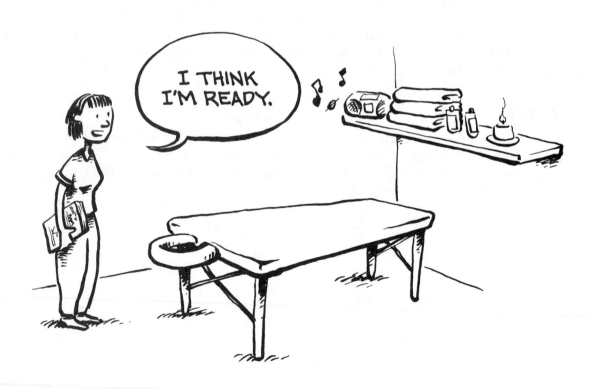

Part 1

Massage Basics

In Part 1, we offer you all the basic information on what massage is today and what benefits it holds for the receiver and giver. You cannot perform a really good massage without a firm grounding in these basics, and your time spent learning this material will be well invested, no matter how far you want to go in the field of massage. You need not become an expert in every point, but you do need at least a basic understanding. The information in Part 1 is the groundwork on which the rest of the book is built. Most important is learning how to see to the comfort of your partner prior to massage and learning to properly perform the massage strokes.

In This Chapter

- ◆ The physiological benefits of massage
- ◆ The psychological benefits of massage
- ◆ The holistic health benefits of massage

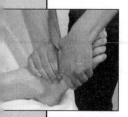 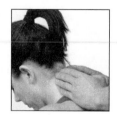 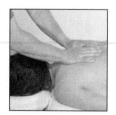 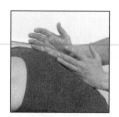 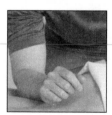 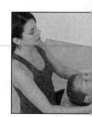

Chapter 1

The Benefits of Massage

The pace of life today creates unrelenting stress for many of us. Stress and the resulting tension and discomfort are reportedly responsible for more than 80 percent of visits to primary care physicians annually. We recognize that stress is unhealthy, but it's difficult to keep up with the numerous demands and deadlines we all face.

That's where massage can help. Through massage, you can relax in a deep and meaningful way and help your body defend against daily stress as well as allow for the rest, repair, and revitalization a balanced body is capable of maintaining in its natural state. Massage is truly holistic; it affects all the body's physical systems—emotional well-being, mental clarity, and connection to the spiritual, however you experience that. Let's take a look at how it works.

The Physiological Effects of Massage

Massage works on all the systems of the body, adjusting them to work in harmony. Consider massage a "tune-up" for your body. From your circulation to your skin to your muscles and bones, you might be surprised at all the parts of your body that can benefit from massage.

The Body Electric

Nerves are the body's "wiring," your electrical system, an incredibly complex biochemical signal system. Signals from the brain constantly course through the spinal cord to all the distant and intricate network of nerves throughout the body. These signals instruct the muscles to relax or contract. When you become tense, your brain sends out too many signals to your muscles to contract, causing them to maintain continuous and unnecessary tension. This puts extra pressure on your bones, tendons, and organs and causes opposing muscles to over-stretch, causing pain.

The muscular system is continuous with the body's connective tissue, linking muscle to muscle. When some muscles tighten, other muscles are forced to tighten to maintain equilibrium, which causes the body to become unbalanced and stiff. When muscles are in such imbalances, joints become misaligned. That sets the stage for degenerative changes such as arthritis. Tightness causes pain, which causes more tension, and you end up with a self-reinforcing cycle of muscle tension and pain.

This is not the body's natural state. Optimally, only muscles actually performing an action should tighten, and all others should remain in a relaxed state. Properly applied, massage helps tight muscles to relax, which relieves unnecessary tension on bones, other muscles, and organs. This, in turn, reduces pain. (We talk more about muscles later in the chapter.)

In the Flow: Circulation

The circulatory system is another important network that runs through the entire body. This network of arteries, capillaries, and veins carries blood throughout the body, feeding every cellular nook and cranny, in many cases paralleling the network of nerves. Blood carries oxygen and food, in the form of glucose, to all the cells in the body. Important but often forgotten is that blood also carries a complex cocktail of hormones that regulate many important bodily functions. Blood carries dissolved minerals important to all organs and systems as well, and it takes away waste products.

Muscular tension, in addition to affecting the larger muscles of the body, tightens the tiny muscles that encircle the blood vessels. This decreases blood flow, especially in the extremities, and increases overall blood pressure. We've heard how harmful high blood pressure can be to our health. Enter massage. Relaxing the muscles through massage reduces constriction in the circulatory system, lowering blood pressure and increasing peripheral circulation. Both are important to good health.

Reducing Energy Constrictions

Some signals move so quickly through the body they can't be attributed to the biochemical activity of the nervous system. The energy system, recognized in Asian and Indian cultures for more than 2,000 years, has only recently been accepted by western medical science.

Lines of energy called meridians run throughtout the body. These meridians, like nerves and blood vessels, have areas that can become constricted, reducing energy flow through an area. Energy flow through the meridians can be improved using acupuncture needles, magnets, or electrical stimulation, but none is as pleasurable as massage.

Definition

In Asian bodywork, the **meridians,** or energy pathways, either start in the head and run down the body toward the feet, or start at the feet and run upward in the body. They follow intricate pathways that correspond to the intersections of muscles groups. Meridians are named for organs, such as the heart, the liver, and the lung, and it is thought that imbalances of energy in the meridians affect the function of the organ systems for which they are named.

Working with Hormones: The Endocrine System

The endocrine system consists of an array of large and small hormone-producing glands throughout the body that produce hormones that affect all the other systems of the body. Examples include insulin, which regulates the level of sugar in the blood, and testosterone, a compelling sex hormone. Until recently, western medical science thought it understood the role of hormones in regulating the body pretty well, but new studies continue to identify new hormones with specific actions (such as obestatin, which controls appetite, discovered in 1995).

The most important hormone for you to know about is adrenaline, secreted by the adrenal glands that sit just above each of your kidneys. When you're under stress, these glands shoot adrenaline into the bloodstream, which causes heart rate to increase, blood pressure to rise, and blood to move to the extremities from our internal organs. This creates a state of hyper-alertness. This heightened state of alertness was useful for our ancestors in "fight-or-flight" situations (when hunting for food—or running to avoid becoming food). But in modern times of unrelenting stress, the adrenal glands tend to produce adrenaline constantly in response to everything from traffic to office deadlines. This always-on response can adversely affect your health.

Back Off _____

When blood is routinely shunted away from the internal organs due to the stress response, chronic digestive problems may result from the impaired circulation. If the heart is forced to beat more rapidly and strongly, it puts extra, unnecessary stress on that vital organ. Extra adrenaline in the system can cause emotional instability and anger. Muscular tension from stress creates pain.

Massage has been shown to reduce the hormone production from the adrenal glands, which can help return them to normal levels of production. In the long run, this can possibly save them from exhaustion, enabling you to have access to adrenaline when you truly need it for emergency situations.

Digestion

Blood carries the food that provides energy in the body's cells, but how does it get into the blood in the first place? That's the digestive system's job. A series of chemical reactions in the stomach and intestines breaks down the food you eat, and the body extracts the nutrients and minerals. These pass through the walls of intestinal capillaries into the blood circulating to all the cells, which carries the nutrients where they're needed.

Proper digestion depends not only on eating the right foods, but also on the muscles that churn food together with digestive juices in the stomach and the muscles that move food through the intestinal system. Just as with the muscles elsewhere in the body, when under stress, these muscles can lose the ability to mechanically digest food, and the body can produce too much or too little of the digestive enzymes used to process food into energy. Relaxing the whole body through massage also relaxes these muscles and enables them to regain proper rhythm.

Press Here _____

The digestive system has more receptor sites to accept neurological signaling chemicals such as adrenaline than does the nervous system. No wonder stress causes so many types of digestive system upset!

Muscles and Bones

We touched on muscles a bit earlier, but let's look at them now in connection with bones. Muscles move the body when you walk, run, swim, write, laugh, and all the other thousands of things you do on a daily basis largely without thinking.

Basically you have two types of muscles in your body: striated and smooth. Striated muscles are typically connected to bones, ligaments, or cartilage and move the parts of the body you can consciously control. Smooth muscles are connected to or surround organs and provide movement that goes on without your conscious control. Both types of muscles are controlled by signals from your brain and spinal cord that are carried by your nerves.

In massage, we focus on the striated muscles, which, together with your bones, comprise your musculoskeletal system. Applying various amounts and types of pressure and movement to those muscles is what the mechanical part of massage is all about.

At Your Fingertips

To practice massage well, you need to know the names of some specific muscles and muscle groups. Spend some time studying the photos in Chapter 4 to learn the names. Consider bookmarking the figures so you can refer to them easily as you're learning strokes that affect specific muscles.

Bones are more than just the rigid structure on which the rest of the body is built. Bones are a part of the connective tissue of the body, a web that's so pervasive that if you were to remove all the body's tissue except the connective tissue, you would still see a recognizable human form. Much of the connective tissue is fascia, thin translucent sheets that surround every specific muscle and each strand of every muscle, the bones, and the organs. It even unites the skin with underlying tissue and bones. Fascia is surprisingly tough and elastic, and when you experience a trauma, it contracts and hardens to protect you. Unfortunately, contracted fascia can exert painful pressure on nerves and blood vessels. Aging, injury, and inactivity can cause the fascia to shorten and thicken. Fortunately, fascia responds well to massage.

Press Here

Ever wonder why babies can put their toes in their mouths easily and many adults can't even bend over and touch their toes? It's because our fascia has shortened and thickened as we have aged.

Bone, the densest form of connective tissue, has a structure much like bamboo, with a hard outer shell and a porous inner marrow to allow for the continuous flow of minerals, fats, and the newborn blood cells that bone marrow produces into and out of the bones. Bones regulate the amount and type of minerals flowing through the bloodstream from moment to moment. In its natural form, bone is a marvel of balanced structure.

Other specific forms of connective tissue include …

◆ Tendons, which are the attachments of muscles to bone.

◆ Ligaments, which attach bones to other bones.

◆ Cartilage, the "gristle" that provides spacing between bones and much greater flexibility and movement than bone—think of your ears.

Many of the painful conditions that develop as we age originate in muscular imbalances that pull the bones into misalignment. When bones are not aligned correctly, wear and tear on the joints and joint capsules can result. This sets the stage for arthritic changes in the joints. Massage can help restore balance between the muscles and prevent or reduce joint damage and dysfunction.

Press Here _____

Cartilage may be thought of in several ways. It might be considered the more flexible parts of bones. Think of your ears and the end of your nose, which are both made of cartridge. The discs between the spinal vertebrae are also cartilage, and as such they may be thought of as spacers and shock absorbers. The ends of bones are coated with yet another form of cartilage which is slick and aids the bones in sliding smoothly against each other when they move, like a Teflon coating.

The Lymphatic System

In addition to blood circulation mentioned earlier, your body has another circulatory system: the lymphatic system. Lymph is a clear or slightly milky fluid that circulates through the lymph vessels and is filtered through the lymph nodes.

The lymphatic system is critical in maintaining your body's fluid balance and in marshalling the immune response against invading bacteria or viral agents. All cells are bathed in lymph fluid. But lymph flow is sluggish because no organ pumps it through the system like the heart pumps blood. Movement and manual action, like massage, enables lymph to have a robust flow and be filtered thoroughly by the lymph nodes.

Press Here _____

Massage is just one part of a healthy body and lifestyle. Drinking plenty of water every day helps keep all systems hydrated, the skin moist, and digestion moving. Drinking lots of water is especially important after you've received a massage because massage pushes wastes from the lymph system into the urinary system. It's a good idea to flush them out as soon as possible.

Breathing Clear: The Respiratory System

Just as your digestive system provides nutrients to your cells through your blood flow, your respiratory system oxygenates your blood. When you inhale, fresh air penetrates tiny air sacs in your lungs, where it moves through porous membranes and makes contact with your blood. There, the red blood cells take in oxygen from the air and are pumped by your heart out to all of the billions of cells in your body. The cells take the food, also carried to them in your blood, and convert the food and oxygen into energy. Then, when you exhale, the waste product, carbon dioxide, is removed.

Massage benefits the respiratory system in numerous ways. When you're relaxed, your breathing slows and deepens, pulling more life-giving air into the system. The relaxation massage provides increases the amount of air lungs can take in and force out. Deep breathing can ease pain, relax tension, and introduce more energy into the body. Deep breaths also massage the chest and abdominal organs from the inside, as the lungs expand and contract rhythmically. Massage of the neck, upper shoulders, and chest areas loosens tightness in those muscles used in the breathing process and allows you to inhale more fully.

If you take a series of short shallow breaths, your nervous system goes on alert and thinks you're facing some danger, so it revs up the production of stress hormones and you begin to feel the sensations of stress, fear, and anxiety in your whole body. Just as short, shallow breaths have a snowball effect on your body's stress reactions, the slowing and deepening of breath during massage calms down your entire system, and your breath gradually deepens and slows even further.

Staying Healthy: The Immune System

We aren't usually aware of the billions of microbes that surround us every day in the air, water, soil, and everything else we come into contact with. Most of these microbes are harmless to us, but among all the harmless ones lurk dangerous ones just looking for a chink in our armor. These disease-causing microbes, whether virus, bacterium, or mold spore, are just waiting for a chance to breach our defenses and make us ill.

The immune system protects us from these relentless attacks. The immune system is made up of white blood cells, antibodies, and numerous other guardians like macrophages, which make up part of the blood and lymph. Antibodies deactivate the invading agents, and the white blood cells devour them. This is a finely tuned system, and it only functions properly when the body is healthy and fit. Unrelieved stress and tension adversely affect the immune system's ability to perform its protective activities. Massage supports a healthy immune response by relieving stress and tension

Skin

Most of us don't think about it this way, but the skin is your largest organ. It seals your vulnerable body from the environment, keeping you warm and moist inside. Its durable surface protects the delicate structures underneath from scrapes and cuts. It regulates your internal temperature through perspiration.

Massage benefits the skin by increasing surface temperature and stimulating blood circulation. It also increases production of natural skin oils by glands in the skin, improving the skin's texture.

Skin health is vitally important to overall health, and massage works to keep skin vital and elastic. Massage oils and lotions increase the skin's moisture and lubricate it during massage.

It's All in Your Mind/Body

The goal of massage is total body relaxation, because a body that's relaxed and in harmony with itself is a healthy body. Just as your brain controls your body by sending out a wide variety of signals through your nervous system, all the parts of your body send signals back to your brain, too. This is a basic feedback system. Your brain needs to know that when it sends a signal, the intended response takes place; the return signal verifies this.

Your body also constantly sends signals to your brain about its overall status, its health, where its parts are in relation to one another, and what is going on within and around it. And unfortunately, many of us ignore the communications from "below" and live in our heads much of the time. Massage allows us to get back "in touch" with what our bodies are telling us.

All Wound Up: Fear, Anxiety, and Stress

A fully relaxed and happy body, in which everything is chugging along as it's supposed to, sends happy and relaxed signals back to the brain. These signals cause the mind to relax, which in turn causes it to send happy and relaxed signals back out to the body, reinforcing the feeling of well-being.

On the flip side, feeling anxious and stressed releases hormonal signals to the body, which tightens up and prepares for "fight or flight" behaviors that in turn send stressful messages back of the brain. This creates a spiraling downward into unpleasant and unsettling physical, emotional, and psychological feelings.

Fear, anxiety, and stress simply can't survive when your built-in feedback system is sending happy, relaxed signals both ways. If you suffer from fear, anxiety, stress, or depression, massage goes a long way toward quelling these feelings and may restore you to a natural balance of good feelings.

Massage as Sleep Aid

Insomnia is a big problem for many people—either they can't get to sleep or they wake up partway through the night and can't get back to sleep. As they lie there awake, the day's concerns come creeping in, and the anxiety, anger, and fear start running replays of all the day's problems.

If you're having trouble sleeping, the reason is usually mental, emotional, or physical. Mental and emotional difficulties are the result of too much fear, anxiety, anger, and stress in your life. Restoring your mind to a natural, relaxed state through massage sometimes eliminates mentally or emotionally created sleep problems.

If you can't sleep because you're feeling physical pain, massage can often help by reducing the pain, so long as it's not caused by an underlying serious medical problem. It's a known medical fact that tension and fear increase the perception of pain, so reducing tension helps you sleep by decreasing your pain level.

But there's good news! Massage, especially in the evening, can help you fall asleep more easily and might help you sleep more soundly through the night. You might even fall asleep during the massage!

Press Here

The amount of sleep you need varies according to the time of year and how hard you're using your body and mind during your waking hours. However long you need some shut-eye, getting enough so you don't really need that afternoon nap is beneficial. Your body needs adequate sleep to perform the downtime maintenance tasks that keep you humming along.

Finding Pleasure in Life and Restoring Your Well-Being

Many people suffer from depression, unable to find pleasure in life. Often people can sink into depression without realizing it, as stresses and strains do their evil work on the body and mind.

Getting back your natural feeling of well-being through massage can cut through depression and bring back the pleasure you can feel in just being alive. Touch is known to be necessary for people of any age; it is a basic pleasure we actively seek from the moment of our birth.

This feeling of well-being is the natural state of the mind and body, but it's frequently lost to the stresses and strains of modern life. Massage can be an important tool in achieving glowing good health and vitality in a busy and challenging life.

At Your Fingertips

Modern life is unnatural, but there are only so many things we can change about it. We can, however, take action and responsibility for our own reactions to stress. Massage is one way we can do that.

How Healthy Do You Want to Be?

Doctors used to be skeptical of the idea that mental disturbance could cause physical problems. However, research and doctors' own personal experiences have convinced many of today's doctors that the so-called psychosomatic illnesses are, indeed, very real.

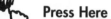

Press Here

Psycho refers to the mind, and *soma* to the body; through complex biochemical interactions, the mind influences the states of wellness or illness in the whole person.

We've all known people who have suffered excessive stress levels and developed stomach and intestinal conditions as a result. Research has shown that a reduction of stress can cause a reduction in the symptoms of ulcers, acid reflux, irritable bowel syndrome (IBS), and Crohn's disease, just to name a few. And mounting evidence shows that some types of cancer are much more common in people with very high stress levels. High blood pressure and associated strokes and heart attacks are related to stress. Numerous other diseases and conditions have similar mind/body links.

Although massage can only address directly the internally generated causes of stress like painful pain-spasm-pain cycles, a person can change how his or her body and mind respond to stress. By reducing negative responses to stress and helping the person achieve a state of natural relaxation, massage can assist in improving a person's overall state of health.

Spiritual Growth

Along with an improvement in physical and mental health, we often see an improvement in what we'll call "spiritual health" in a person who has been getting massages. Regardless of what if any religion you follow, you'll realize that there's more to life than just the physical body and brain and their reactions. The nonphysical, or metaphysical, can be equally important to a healthy and balanced person.

By putting the physical, mental, and emotional states in harmony, massage can open the door to spiritual growth and awareness. You might find a realization of your personal connection to all things as a natural effect of massage. Human connection is a part of spirituality, and the connection of massaging a friend's hand or shoulders to soothe her anxiety and tension, calming a distressed or distracted child with soothing strokes, or expressing concern and care to an aging parent through touch might help make you aware of the power of caring connection.

Increased Intimacy

Although anyone can use this book to learn massage, we have thought particularly of couples when writing it. The touching, stroking, rubbing, and other connections made between two people during a massage can go a long way toward opening doors to greater levels of intimacy. If the spark has gone out of a relationship, massage can often rekindle the flame. Massage can be beneficial in different ways between parents and children and friends as well.

It's important to note that the positive effects of massage for the recipient are only half the story. It is well recognized that most of us feel better about ourselves when we're able to help others. In an early scientific study of the effects of massage on premature infants, the massaged infants gained weight much more quickly and were released from the hospital on average 5 days sooner than their nonmassaged peers. The massaged infants also showed numerous other measurable signs of thriving. The volunteer "grandmothers" who performed the massage showed lowered blood pressure and pulse, increased relaxation response, and an increase in endorphins, the "feel-good" hormones.

Massage positively affects us in all areas of our life, from our mental, emotional, and spiritual selves to the workings of our body's systems all the way down to the cellular level. It even helps us reach beyond the limits of our selves to reach out in connection with others. Through touch we can re-establish balance in our various mind and body systems that may allow us to live in a state of enhanced well-being.

The Least You Need to Know

- ◆ Massage relaxes, and relaxation is beneficial to your physical, psychological, and overall (holistic) health.
- ◆ Massage helps all the body's interrelated systems work optimally at their specific tasks and stay in proper balance with one another.
- ◆ Massage is useful in preventing or assisting in the healing of numerous *dis-ease* conditions.

In This Chapter

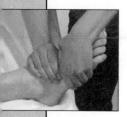
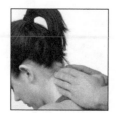
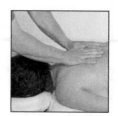
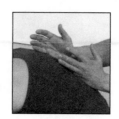
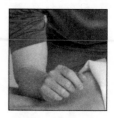
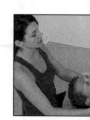

Setting Up

Now that you know all the benefits massage can bring, you might be eager to grab your partner and get some hands-on work. Before you do, though, do yourself (and your partner) a favor and read this chapter.

A little advance planning and consideration of where you're going to give the massage, what if any lubricants you'll use, and how and where you'll ask your partner to position his body will make the massage that much more pleasurable for both of you.

The Environment

For massage to be effective, maximum comfort is essential. The room in which you give your massages is very important. It must make your partner feel completely at ease, completely private and secure. A small room is more cozy and intimate-feeling than a really large room, although your room choices will obviously be limited by what's available to you.

Massage reduces your receiver's pulse and blood pressure, and blood will bathe the internal organs in a relaxed state. This reduces the blood flow to the arms and legs and your partner can get chilly, so it's important that the room be warm enough that your partner is comfortable and able to relax, not think about how she wished she'd worn a pair of socks. For most people, 73° to 75° Fahrenheit should be warm enough, although check with your partner now and then to be sure she's not too cool. Seldom will you hear that your partner is too warm, although you might feel warm when she is comfortable, especially while you're working. If you're worried about getting too warm, dress in lightweight clothing.

Back Off

You want your partner to be cozy and feel secure, but if you're working in a cramped space, you might find yourself in awkward positions as you work around your partner. Try to create space for massage where you can take a wide stance when needed or have room for a chair for the parts of massage that are best done seated.

Indirect, low-level lighting is more relaxing than bright overhead lights. If the room has overhead lighting, turn it off! That harsh brightness will disturb the serene mood you want to create and will shine in your partner's eyes when she's supine (face up). Low-wattage lamps—or better yet, scented candles—provide a more restful environment. In addition, if your partner lacks some confidence about how her body looks, she won't want harsh, glaring lights that highlight every flaw. The cliché that a woman looks better by candlelight has some truth to it. Opt for softer, more flattering light.

Back Off

Avoid fluorescent lamps, whether overhead or elsewhere, as they have an almost imperceptible flicker that can produce headaches, eyestrain, and other ailments. Sometimes they buzz, too. None of this is conducive to a relaxing and healing atmosphere.

They say "Music hath charm to sooth the savage breast." Although we doubt you'll massage many savages, we do think music can be important in establishing a soothing mood for the massage session. Just be sure you play music that has the desired effect on both of you.

Music you like just might be making your partner grit her teeth—generally not what a relaxed person does. The pace of the music shouldn't be too fast because you'll tend to work to the tempo of the music. Rapid massage strokes are not relaxing. Many find that classical or baroque music produces the desired effect, while others prefer New Age or other soothing instrumental music. Instrumental songs are often best to go with rather than songs with distracting lyrics. Most of us need to turn our verbal selves off for a while so we can focus on the pleasurable sensations of the body. Whatever works for the two of you is the right music.

At Your Fingertips

Keep the volume relatively soft. You want it loud enough to hear easily and block out background noise, but not loud enough to distract either of you.

Even if you're exceptionally good friends, your partner probably will want to be at least partially covered to avoid becoming chilled as she relaxes. We've found that ordinary bed linens and towels are the best things to use for draping. Full-size sheets work well; they give you plenty of fabric to layer and provide warmth. Twin fitted sheets fit a massage table perfectly, and flat twin sheet are just right for a single-layer drape. A lightweight fleece blanket over the top sheet offers an extra layer that can be removed or added according to your partner's preference, which might change during the massage. Some people prefer to use thick terry towels for warmth. You'll need the large ones sometimes called bath sheets or beach towels. There are no hard-and-fast rules about what to use for draping. Use whatever provides the amount of privacy and warmth to keep your friend comfortable.

Back Off

Draping with something too large invites fabric to trail onto the floor where it could get dirty or possibly trip you, so avoid grossly oversized drapes.

It's best to use 100 percent cotton fabrics for draping. (High-polyester-content sheets feel like what they are—plastic.) Some people are allergic to other types of fabric, and cotton affects few people. Cotton fabrics are also easy to keep clean with regular washing can be sanitized with bleach if necessary.

It's useful to have a few pillows close at hand as well to help your partner get comfortable:

◆ A pillow to bolster under the knees in face-up (supine) position takes pressure off her lower back.

◆ A pillow under her ankles when she's face down (prone) makes her feet more comfortable.

◆ A pillow under her head when she's lying on her side and another between her knees and ankles keeps her joints neutral and padded.

A "huggy" pillow to support the top arm when your partner's lying on her side makes the finishing touch for a truly nurturing position.

Avoid Interruptions

Find a time when you're least likely to be interrupted, and maybe even put a "Do Not Disturb" sign on the door before you begin the massage. If you have a cell phone in your pocket or purse, turn it off or put it on mute. If a regular telephone is nearby, switch off the ringer or set it to go directly to voicemail without ringing first. Send the kids to Grandma's for the night.

In other words, do everything you can to ensure quiet during the time you've set aside for the massage.

At Your Fingertips

Massage moves waste products out of your lymph and blood and through your kidneys. Drinking plenty of liquid during the day is important to maintaining the fluid and electrolyte balances in your system. It's even more important to drink plenty of fluids after a massage so your body can dilute toxic waste and flush it out of your system.

Lubricants: What to Use and Where to Get It

The purpose of a lubricant is to reduce friction on the skin and allow your hands to move smoothly during the massage. Lubricants can be liquid (lotions, creams, or oils) or solid (powders).

Because of the popularity of massage, many commercial products are available, but you might want to experiment with simple lubricants like a light olive oil—it worked for the ancient Greeks and Romans! If you use vegetable oil, be sure it's a type that doesn't easily go rancid at room temperature. Be careful with some nut oils, though. Many people are deathly allergic to nuts, especially peanut, so avoid this if your partner has a nut allergy. But some people are allergic to other nut oils, too, including coconut oil.

It might be best to use a commercial lubricant to be safe from any nut allergies, such as any of the creams, lotions, oils or gels from Biotone, Massage Fx, Bon Vital, Touch Essentials, and Soothing Touch, but be sure to check the ingredients list and avoid nut oils if your receiver tells you she has such an allergy. In Appendix A, we give you a list of sources for commercial lubricants.

Back Off

Although you might be tempted to use ordinary mineral oil or mineral oil–based "baby oil," don't. Mineral oil clings to the skin and clogs the pores, preventing the elimination of toxins through the skin. Mineral oil is absorbed through the skin, too, and the liver has to detox it before it's eliminated. As it moves through your body, the mineral oil picks up fat-soluble vitamins and strips them from your system. If you've been using a mineral oil–based oil on your baby, please stop. Plenty of safe vegetable oil alternatives are available to use instead. Always check labels for ingredients before buying lubricants.

Most people prefer a lotion or cream lubricant. These products provide slickness as you first apply them, work in without leaving greasy residue on the sheets, and generally don't ruin your sheets. Many people don't like to feel oily after a massage, and for these people, it's best to use lotions or creams that are fully absorbed.

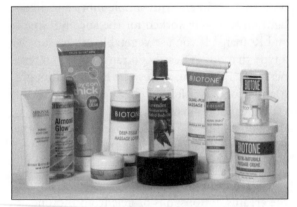

Here are some examples of commercial lubricants you can buy to make your massages silky smooth and comfortable.

Men with profuse and coarse body hair and anyone whose skin breaks out from oil-based lubricants might want to experiment with powder. If you try working with powder, look for basic baby powder with a cornstarch base rather than talc. Some people are allergic to talc, and questions have been raised over its safety even for people not allergic to it. There's often a 12- to 24-hour delay before allergic symptoms to lubricants appear.

In most parts of the country, you can find massage creams and lotions in health food stores and some cosmetic supply shops. If you can't find what you want locally, you can get just about anything online or by mail order these days, and lubricants are no exception. Check out the ads in massage and health magazines. Also check the resources listed in Appendix A for some suppliers.

Massage Tables and Other Options

If you have the space and want to, you can certainly devote an area of your home specifically to massage. If you're like most people, though, you probably don't have space in your home for a full-time massage area. A portable folding massage table might be just the thing for you. Folding massage tables set up quickly and can be easily folded so you can carry or store them between sessions in a small space such as under the bed or in a closet. (Check out Appendix A for some sources for tables.)

When selecting a folding massage table, be sure to find one that's very sturdy and substantial when it's set up. Be certain the table is rated to support the heaviest person you're likely to have lying on it.

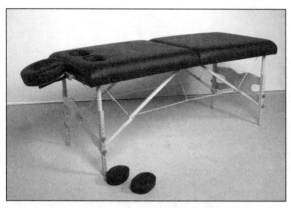

A professional massage table.

When you first start massaging, you might want to do without a massage table and instead work on a mat on the floor. Mats primarily for Thai massage or shiatsu work fine for massage, too, (see Appendix A). If you're considering a mat, get one that's large enough that you can kneel on it while performing the massage; you can also find mat systems that come with a separate kneeling pad. A mat on the floor works fine for many types of massage but can be limiting and harder on the person giving the massage. Experiment and find out what works best for you and your partner.

![hand icon] **Back Off**

> When your partner gets on the table, be sure she doesn't sit right in the middle of the table, because that's the weakest part. Have her sit more toward one end. This distributes more of the weight onto the table legs for greater stability and security.

Be sure whatever surface you have your receiver on is neither too high nor too low for you to work comfortably. Check out how you're standing when you're giving the massage. Are you bending at the waist and experiencing low back pain? If so, the surface is too low. If your neck and shoulders become uncomfortable from lifting your shoulders up toward your ears, the supporting surface is too high.

To determine the proper table height, stand at the side of the table with your arm hanging down at your side. The backs of your fingers should just rest on the table with your wrist straight. This is simply a starting point, and you may need to adjust the table up or down a notch as necessary.

The Massage Positions

When you picture someone getting a massage, you probably picture the receiver in the prone, or face-down position. This position provides good access to the back and the backs of the legs. A pillow or bolster under the lower legs helps to keep the receiver's feet from cramping and makes this position more comfortable. It's also the most uncomfortable position for some people, so check with your partner about her preferences. People with chronic low back pain may not be able to lie comfortably in the prone position. Others will experience stuffy noses immediately when they are face down.

Prone position should not be used for neck massage. If you don't have a massage table with an adjustable face cradle, it'll be very difficult to position your partner so her neck doesn't get uncomfortable too quickly. You can use rolled towels to help with this problem when working on a mat on the floor, but it can still be problematic. The Comfort Mat System includes a face cradle so the receiver's head doesn't have to be turned to the side, which puts uncomfortable stress on the neck.

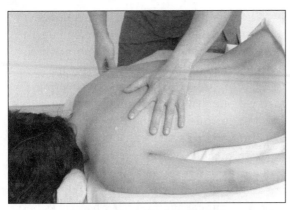

The prone position for massage.

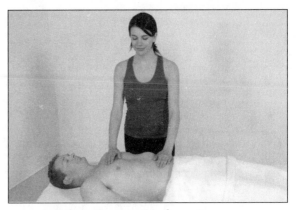

The supine position for massage.

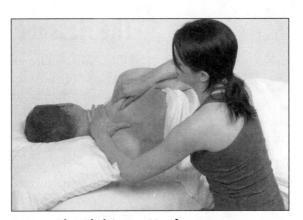

The side-lying position for massage.

Having your partner face up (supine) on a massage table or the floor allows you to massage the head, face, neck, shoulders, fronts and backs of the arms, the abdomen, legs, and feet. The supine position has numerous benefits, and most people can be comfortable lying on their backs. You can even work on portions of the back and hips while your partner is in the supine position. Many people feel more comfortable being able to look at their surroundings and the person who is massaging them. Some people need a pillow under their head for comfort when they're lying on their back, and a pillow under the knees takes strain off the lower back.

An often-overlooked position is the side-lying position. With a pillow supporting your receiver's head, another in her arms, and a third between her flexed knees and ankles, she'll be in a very comfortable position. You can work her neck, shoulders, back, hips, legs, and feet in this position. The only downside is that you have to be especially careful of your own body mechanics, as working on someone in this position can be somewhat awkward.

You don't always have to work with a massage table or with your partner lying down. You can give massage with your partner sitting on a chair. This works best with a sturdy, narrow chair without arms. You can have your receiver sit normally in the chair to massage her lower legs and feet. For back, shoulder, neck, arm, and hand massage, have your friend sit backward in the chair so her legs straddle the chair seat. Have her lean forward against a pillow and have some more pillows on the tabletop the chair is up against so she can rest her arms on the table and her head on the pillows.

Generally, when you massage a seated person, he'll be clothed, so draping is not an issue.

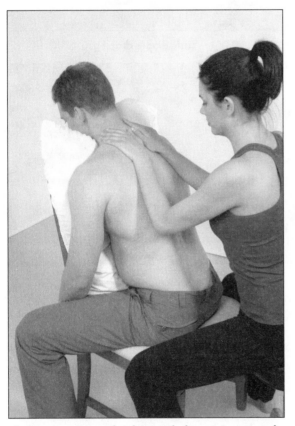

Some massage can be done with the receiver seated.

In the following chapters, we give you detailed instructions for each type of massage, so follow our lead, experiment, and settle on what works best for you and your partner.

Covering Up

We briefly touched on draping earlier in the chapter in the setup section. Here, we give you more specific tips on draping your partner.

> **At Your Fingertips**
>
> It's nice to have a twin-size sheet to cover your partner, with a fleece blanket or bath sheet over the sheet. This enables you to adjust the covers to warm or cool the receiver.

Draping the receiver in the supine position is pretty straightforward.

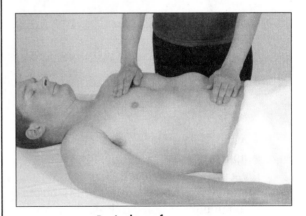

Basic drape for a man.

For certain areas, you'll use special draping. For instance, when you're working on the right arm, that's the only area of the receiver's body that needs to be uncovered—unless she's too warm and wants her other arm or perhaps her feet and lower legs uncovered.

You can use two basic draping methods for the receiver's legs:

◆ You can simply push the cover over and tuck it beneath the leg you aren't massaging so you have access to the other leg and thigh.

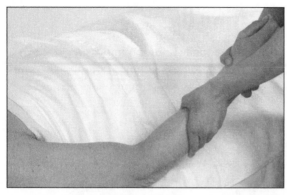

The basic drape.

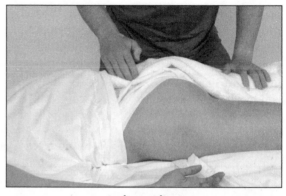

Basic diaper draping.

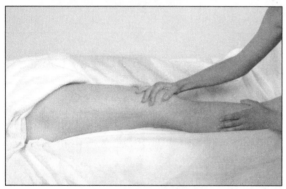

The simple leg drape.

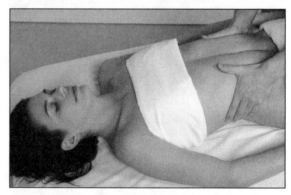

The pillowcase drape.

◆ For the "diaper drape," start as with the simple drape, but bring the drape *under* the leg you're massaging. The receiver might even hold the section you've pulled through under her leg to keep the drape more secure and provide modesty, particularly if she has removed all her clothing under the cover. This is also a good drape to use if you're going to perform joint mobilization movements with the legs.

If you're going to work on the abdomen, you might want to provide a breast drape for women, which can be as simple as a folded pillowcase to cover the chest area.

You could also use a "surgical drape," which is a way of positioning the cover sheet to expose the abdomen while keeping the breasts covered. Essentially, you pull the middle of the draping sheet over to one side to expose the abdomen, and tuck the sheet in under her body to hold it in place.

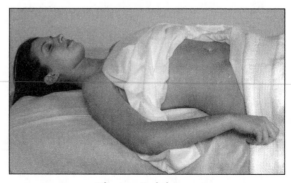

The surgical drape.

Draping for the prone position is not much different from draping for the supine position. The backs of the receiver's legs can be draped in the same way as the front of her legs were draped in the supine position. Generally, no arm or neck massage is done while the receiver is in the prone position, so you only have her back and legs to drape. It's straightforward, though. Just fold the drape down to hip level.

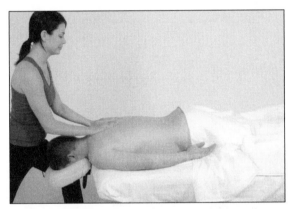

Basic draping for the prone position.

Draping to protect the receiver's modesty in the side-lying position is a little more challenging than other positions. If you start from the supine position with the receiver's leg already draped in a diaper drape, you could place a pillow under her head, place another between her knees and ankles, and give her a third pillow to hug.

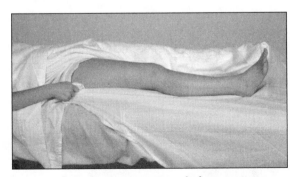

Starting from the supine position before turning onto the side.

Then, have her turn away from you on the table or floor mat as you hold the drape

covering her lower back in place. This draping gives you nice access to the whole side of her body. You can use a heat pack or small pillow to help secure the drape at her lower back, or you may slide the drape between her hip and the table.

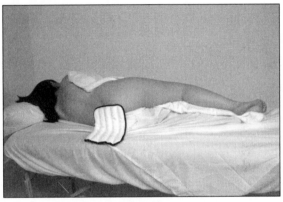

Draping after turning on the side.

Your understanding of some basic comfort measures such as lubricant use and draping procedures during a massage makes the experience more comfortable. It's also important to set the stage and create a private, warm environment in which your partner can relax completely with gentle lighting and quiet music. These comfort measures help insure an enjoyable massage experience.

The Least You Need to Know

- ◆ The comfort of the massage environment is critical to the overall massage experience.
- ◆ Proper use of lubricants is important to a successful massage.
- ◆ Although a massage table is best, you can do massage successfully with a massage mat on the floor or even with your partner sitting in a chair.
- ◆ Draping is important to preserve the receiver's modesty and also to provide extra warmth.

In This Chapter

- ◆ The prepared partner
- ◆ Limbering exercises
- ◆ Self-care and body mechanics
- ◆ Breathing and energy

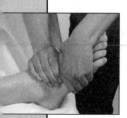
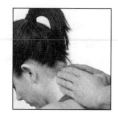
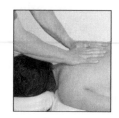
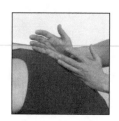
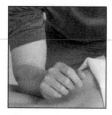
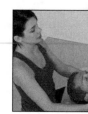

Preparation for Massage

Before you think of giving someone else a massage, you should consider whether you have the physical strength and stamina to perform a vigorous hour or more session or even just a gentle 30-minute massage. (Most people are healthy enough for this level of exertion, but check with your doctor if you have any health concerns that might give you pause about the exertion of performing a massage.) Giving and receiving massage improves your strength and stamina as you play with it, and improves your overall health and vitality with its effects.

In this chapter, we give you tips on physical warm-up: stretches and other premassage exercises you can do to get ready. We also share information on the other kinds of preparation, including breathing and talking with your partner to get the best massage possible.

Warming Up and Getting Limber

Giving a massage is exercise, and just like you'd warm up before a run or a workout at the gym, you should warm up before you give someone a massage. Although you'll use your whole body when massaging your partner, the brunt of the effort flows through your shoulders, chest, hands, and arms, so it's important to loosen up your upper body before a massage.

The following exercises help warm up your upper body and prepare your body for giving massage. They might also help you maintain a higher level of comfort in your upper body if you perform them regularly. These make excellent stretches to do with your partner, too, before a massage or anytime. Simply perform them facing your partner.

Be sure to move only to the point of comfortable stretch, flirting with the edges of your limits of flexibility; it's counterproductive to try to stretch past your limits. Lengthen your body on the inhalations, and sink slightly deeper into the stretch on the exhalations.

1. Standing, with length in the front of your body and with your shoulders low and broad, place your palms together in front of your heart. This is the heart salutation. Hold for two or three deep breaths. (Hold all the stretches this long.)

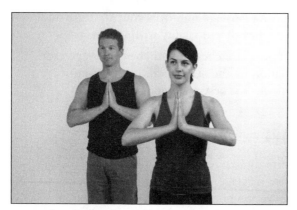

Begin by standing and placing your palms together.

2. Sweep your arms down to your sides as you exhale.

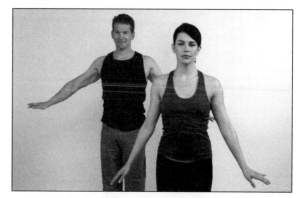

Bring your arms to your sides.

3. Then, inhale as you raise your arms over your head strongly. Keep your shoulders low; don't allow them to come up toward your ears.

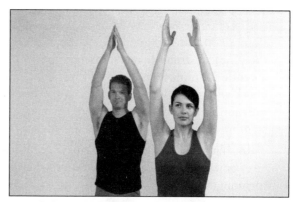

Inhale as you raise your arms over your head.

4. Bring your forearms together. Hold for two or three deep breaths.

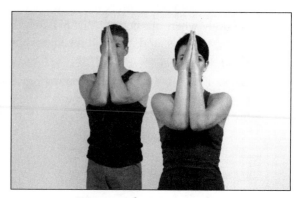

Bring your forearms together.

5. Keeping your shoulders low and your chest open, bring your hands downward so your palms are together in front of your heart, with a straight line from elbow to elbow. Hold.

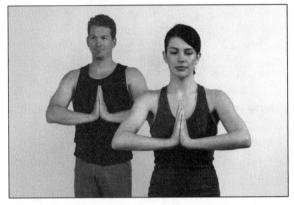

Bring your palms together in front of your heart.

6. Move your hands to the left and hold, making sure to keep your left elbow low. Take a few breaths. Repeat on the right side.

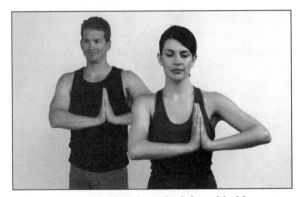

Move your hands to the left and hold.

7. Rotate your fingers forward (your palms should still be together). Hold and then rotate them back so your fingers are pointing toward your heart. Hold.

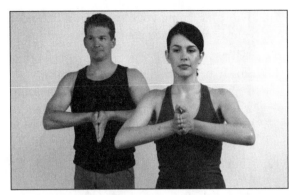

Rotate your hands away from your torso and then toward your heart.

8. Lace your fingers together, and rotate your hands so your palms are facing forward.

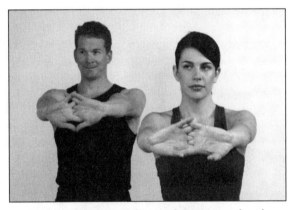

Lace your fingers together, and rotate your hands.

9. With your fingers still laced together, inhale as you raise your arms overhead again, your palms facing up.

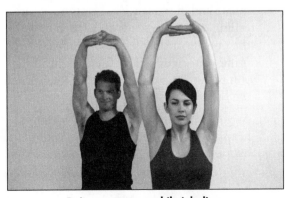

Raise your arms while inhaling.

10. This time, bring your arms down behind your back and lace your fingers together again.

11. Slowly bring your clasped hands away from your back, and lean forward, bending at the hips, not rounding your upper back. It helps to think about leading with your chest. Hold for several breaths.

12. After you return your arms to your sides, bring your left arm straight across your chest.

13. With your right hand, pull your left arm in closer to your chest. This intensifies the stretch between your shoulder blades. Hold for a few breaths and then repeat on the right side.

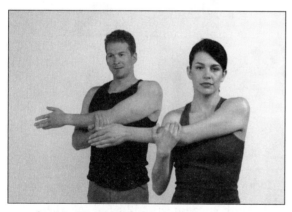

This move intensifies the stretch between your shoulder blades.

14. Standing with your legs fairly far apart, inhale and lift your right arm toward the ceiling as you stretch your left arm down the outside of your left leg. Gradually bring your right arm farther overhead so you're getting a nice side bend. Repeat on the other side.

15. As you inhale, bring your right arm overhead and place your right hand on the back of your neck.

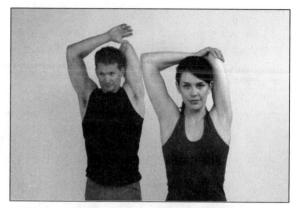

Bring your right arm over your head and then put your hand on the back of your neck.

16. Reach up with your left hand, and pull your right elbow in closer to your head. Take your left arm behind your back and reach up toward the right hand with your left hand. Don't be discouraged if you can't grasp your hands together—it's a difficult move. Just feel the stretch, breathe into it, and repeat on the opposite side.

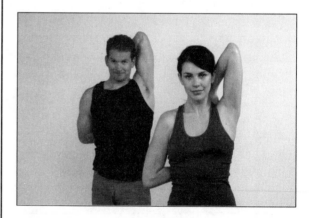

The more you do this one, the more flexible you'll become.

17. Finally, inhale and raise your arms overhead and then out to the sides as you "swan dive" forward, bending at your hips, with a straight spine. Then fold and hang loosely from your hips. If you can get your fingertips or palms to the floor, all the better.

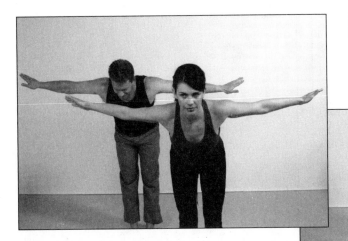

Swan dive forward. If you can touch the floor, so much the better.

After this, you should be completely loose and limber and ready to go.

18. Slowly roll back to an upright standing position.

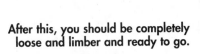

Press Here

Yoga movements can go a long way toward improving both strength and flexibility. Twisting at the waist, and front, back, and side bends are excellent for giving your torso flexibility. Correctly executed forward bends strengthen the upper back muscles between the shoulder blades that are especially important for healthy posture while giving massage. For more information on yoga, see *The Complete Idiot's Guide to Yoga Illustrated, Fourth Edition* (Alpha Books, 2006).

Taking Care of *You*

Massage can be a physically demanding activity. You won't injure your body if you use it properly, but it is possible to hurt yourself if you don't pay attention to *body mechanics* and self-care. This is especially true if you do other activities that are hard on your hands, arms, shoulders, and back like gardening, computer work, construction, bicycling, or stocking shelves, just to name a few.

Definition

Body mechanics is the term used to describe how you hold and move your body during the massage, and it's just as important as your health. Not using proper body mechanics can harm your body during massage, resulting in aches and pains.

When you learn good self-care and body mechanics and practice them while you massage, you can create body habits that benefit you in your work life, hobbies, and sports. When you establish good form in massage, your whole body feels better—you feel more balanced and you're more likely to be pain free, especially if your partner has been massaging you as well! The more you use balanced alignment during massage, the more likely you are to become more flexible and graceful.

Practicing Good Body Mechanics

Taking proper care of your own body is important to anyone who wishes to give massages. If you're not feeling well, you can't apply the necessary energy and concentration. In this section, we offer some tips on how to give a massage so you benefit your partner as well as yourself.

Keep all your joints in line. This means your wrist and elbows aren't sticking out in different directions, but are slightly flexed. Aim for a nice, straight line from your shoulder to fingertips. Your shoulders and torso should be aiming in the direction of your stroke. Your head should be balanced on your upright neck. Even your hips should be facing in the direction of the stroke so you're not bent around like a pretzel. Keep an upright spine; don't lean forward at the waist or your partner might have to work out back spasms when it's her turn to massage you! Bend your knees when you need to be lower; this is the exception to the rule of keeping your joints aligned.

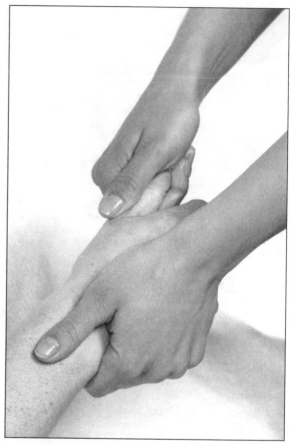

All your joints need to be in good alignment.

At Your Fingertips

If you have hyper-mobile joints in your thumbs, fingers, or wrists—meaning they bend back farther than those of most people you know—be sure to use your other hand to support your working hand.

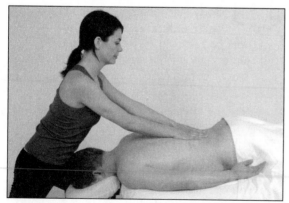

Good form is important in giving a massage so you don't harm yourself.

Have your strokes come from your whole body. Your legs are stronger than your arms; use them to propel a stroke up through your torso, through your shoulders, and down through your arms and hands and you won't tire as quickly. If you combine this principle with keeping your joints in line, you can see how using the whole body makes your massage movements more fluid.

Besides preventing repetitive strain injuries, doing massage this way has a much more connected feel than if you do the same stroke just using your hands and arms.

Try it for yourself. Make some of the flowing strokes in Chapter 4 with your partner both using your whole, well-aligned body and then using just your arms and hands. Ask your partner how each stroke feels different.

Press Here

Massage at its best is a dance, and as in a dance, the whole aligned body is in constant fluid movement. Just as having the movements of massage come from your whole body makes the massage feel more connected, moving your body constantly with your strokes is another way of making your strokes feel more connected for your partner, and you will feel less tired after the massage.

Your Hands: Your Most Important Asset

Few things in this world are as satisfying and beautiful as your own hands providing pleasure and relaxation to someone. The condition of your hands and nails is one of the most important things in giving a massage. Smooth hands feel delightful, while rough hands with ragged cuticles can be aggravating and uncomfortable. Besides making it more comfortable for your partner, the sensitivity in your hands and your experience of their smooth skin will be enhanced.

If your work or other activities are hard on your hands, consider wearing gloves. Scissors, emery boards, and products like salt glows (coarse salt in an essential oil base, often scented), hand brushes, and sugar or microdermabrasion scrubs can smooth out roughness and reduce ragged cuticles.

Pay daily attention to your hands. The more massage you do, the more you'll recognize and appreciate the miracle of your hands' dexterity. Being mindful helps you avoid cuts that can be sore when you give massage. Taking care of your cuticles helps avoid painful hangnails, too.

Practicing Good Form

You don't need to stare down at your hands and the body you're massaging all the time to know what's happening during a massage. Your neck will hurt if you are always looking at your hands. Your back will hurt, too, if you bend over at the waist to observe what your hands are doing.

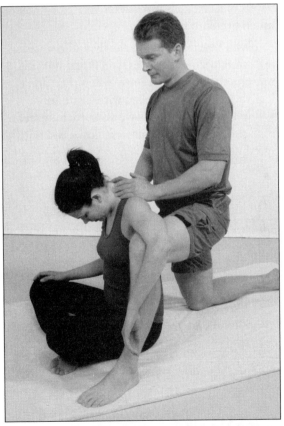

Keeping your head upright while giving a massage is very important to good form.

Try closing your eyes and allowing your hands to be your eyes. You might find it's easier to keep an upright posture this way. Or it might be helpful to look across the room or out a window to maintain good neck and back posture—if you can do it without losing your focus on the partner's body. We humans tend to be very vision oriented, while massage is about touch and movement. Your eyes are in your hands during massage.

Easy Does It

The "no pain, no gain" adage has no place in massage. Finesse beats force every time. You can have an effect deep in your partner's muscles without pushing or working hard. Perceived depth of a stroke is not always related to how much pressure you apply.

If you practice sinking slowly and consciously into your partner's tissues, you'll feel how his muscles melt and turn loose when they don't feel they're being attacked with brute force. Using brute force can leave your partner feeling sore and beaten up. It also can leave you with numbness, tingling, or pain in your wrists and hands.

> **At Your Fingertips**
>
> As with life, variety is the spice of massage. Your partner will enjoy massages more when you use a variety of strokes applied in different areas. Massage actually can get boring if you do the same things over and over. More important, you are likely to experience symptoms of repetitive strain injury if you don't use a variety of strokes. With variety, everybody wins.

Going Slowly

We live in a deadline-driven, 24/7 society, and not many of us are rewarded for doing anything

slowly. Massage is an exception. When you're learning to massage, you'll tend to start out too fast. Learn to slow down—way down. Don't worry about going too slowly; it's difficult to massage too slowly.

> **Press Here**
>
> The body responds to slow, graceful massage strokes by entering into what's called a *parasympathetic state*, the opposite of the fight-or-flight response.

Avoid playing music with a fast tempo while you're giving a massage, as it will drive you to massage faster. Breathe slowly and smoothly, ideally in sync with your partner, and your slow, deliberate strokes will put her into a relaxed state of bliss.

Getting Centered and Grounded

Before beginning a massage, it's important that you be centered and grounded. Being centered means being focused in the moment, calm and at peace, the day's concerns left somewhere else.

Breathing exercises can help bring you into the present. Deep breathing and full exhalations oxygenate your blood and expel toxins, leaving you feeling energized but calm. Your calm will radiate out from you as you massage your partner, helping her feel calm and fully relaxed. She'll experience your calm and focus as deep and satisfying. You'll be able to respond well to her needs and preferences during the massage when you are fully present.

It's important to ground yourself before you start your massage. Many of us spend most of our time totally in our heads. It really helps to be in your body before you start massaging someone else's body. As with centering, grounding requires you to be in the moment. Start by feeling the floor supporting your body. Notice the alignment and ease (or lack of it) you're feeling in your body right now. Close your eyes and experience fully all the sensations of your breath.

 Back Off

> Don't skip the step of grounding yourself before you give someone a massage. Being grounded in your own body while you do massage helps you avoid performing actions that could cause you discomfort later.

Focusing on Breathing and Energy

Energy and breath are like two sides of the same coin. In a state of health, life energy flows freely through the body in a balanced manner and contributes to vitality. Disrupted, disorganized, or depleted energy makes a person feel unwell or tired.

Definition

> By **energy**, we mean the life force that is within each one of us.

Breathing is the most immediate and essential ingredient of energy. We could go a few days without water and possibly a few weeks without food, but we can't go for 2 minutes without air. We naturally manipulate our energy through breath in many ways. We become breathless with excitement and hold our breath in fear. We sigh with relief, yawn in boredom, gasp in surprise. All these responses naturally fill immediate needs for oxygen and energy in the body.

Stress often contributes to shallow breathing, which disrupts optimal energy in the body, but controlled deep breathing helps us transform the air we breathe into energy. The oxygenation of our cells produces inner energy that radiates throughout the body. This energy can be used for anything, but here we'll focus on massage, a most effective and wonderful use for it. Having this vibrant inner energy can physically fuel the action and effort you exert while you're massaging your partner. When you're overflowing with the vital energy from full breath, you'll have plenty of energy to share with your partner.

Energy and breath, used with intention, can take the pleasure and relaxation of a good massage to a whole new level. You can use shared breathing patterns to increase personal connection with your partner. You can help your partner relax by suggesting, either verbally or by exaggerating the depth of your own breath, that she slow and deepen her breath. Or you can help your partner raise a flagging energy level by encouraging a strong, deep, and more rapid breathing pattern.

Press Here

> You might find that your breath naturally gets in sync with your partner's breath during these exercises. If it doesn't, it might mean your breathing rates are just very different.

Getting in touch with your partner's breath and energy before you begin to massage helps connect the two of you and gives you a sense for what feels good to her during her massage. You'll be more likely to notice if she holds her breath, which might indicate discomfort, and feel the release of tension with her long and satisfied sigh. When you're aware of breath and energy, you'll be more sensitive to her responses to your touch.

The Prepared Partner

You can't give what you don't have, and during a massage, you'll want to give your partner all the health-promoting energy you can. Get enough rest so when you give massage you'll be alert to your partner's needs and to how your own body is responding to the activity. Being fully awake helps you remember to apply good body mechanics as well.

Press Here

Eat, drink, and be merry. High-quality nutrition, plenty of fresh water, and exercise help the body function smoothly and recover from strain. Have fun. A positive attitude supports your body and your mind.

Developing self-awareness is your best protection from injury. Fortunately, if you and your partner are both giving each other massage, it's one of the best ways to develop good body consciousness. If you are attuned to the signals your body constantly sends you, you'll be able to modify massage techniques when they begin to cause you discomfort. Listen to your body; it will tell you when you are using it healthfully— and when you're not.

At Your Fingertips

When you're giving a massage, you are close to your partner, and often to her nose. Being clean and smelling nice is just part of creating a pleasant environment. Unless you have both had onions or other strong-smelling foods before a massage, you might want to consider not only brushing your teeth, but having some strong breath mints as well.

As a receiver, it's nice to bathe before your massage. One of your skin's roles in life is to remove some bodily wastes through perspiration. You'll want to be clean so these waste products and the soil from daily living are not rubbed into your skin. Most of the lubricants we recommend are good for your skin, and it's beneficial to leave them on after your massage.

Premassage Q&A

Before you lay a hand on your partner, talk to her. Find out how she's feeling. Has her day been demanding and stressful? Did she have a particularly vigorous racquetball game in the afternoon, and now has sore muscles as a result? Does she have a cut or bruise that would be painful to touch or another recent injury you should be aware of?

These types of questions can set the stage for your massage. The answers to questions you ask give you valuable information about what kind of massage your partner desires, and whether particular areas of her body will require extra attention or need to be avoided.

Many of us live in our heads so much that until someone asks specific questions about how we're feeling, we're not very aware of how we're doing. We might be totally unaware we've been clinching our jaws in stress and anger during the day. We might not have noticed that our backs and necks are sore from hours at the computer. You can ask your partner to scan her body for you, to try and feel where anything is uncomfortable or feeling tight. It's often helpful for the person to move around a bit while scanning for problem areas.

Hopefully, you know your partner well enough to be aware of any significant health challenges she might have. If she's suffering from any illnesses or conditions that make you unsure whether you should give her a massage, it's always best to err on the side of caution and have her check with her doctor.

Back Off

If your partner has the sniffles, ask if she might be coming down with a cold. A cold, fever, or other whole-body infection is already putting stress on the immune system, and in this case, it would be best to delay the massage until the cold is almost gone. At that point, massage might hasten it out of the body; but especially at the beginning of a cold or flu, massage is likely to make the condition worse.

In some cases, you might not even need to ask your partner questions about how she's feeling. You might notice she's favoring one leg when she walks or is unconsciously rubbing her right shoulder. You might see facial expressions that suggest worry, stress, or tired lines around her eyes. It's never a bad idea to confirm how your partner is feeling. You might be amazed that your partner is often unaware of the shoulder she is rubbing, the hand pressed to her lower back, or the slight limp. Most of us are pleased when someone is paying enough attention to notice these things, and even more pleased when relief in the form of massage is forthcoming.

Sometimes your partner will want just certain areas massaged, and frequently she will have preferences about the amount of pressure. Ask specific questions, because this is *her* massage, and it should be the way she wants and needs it, not how you'd like to have a massage for yourself. Massaging as we like to be massaged is probably the simplest and most common error we make. Tailor the massage you give to as many of her specific requests as you can, and it will be a wonderful massage!

Intention

Your premassage conversation will establish even before the massage that it's your intention to provide a customized special massage for your partner. Whether it's your intention to reduce discomfort in specific tired muscles, give nurturing care to a grieving friend, or ease away the stress that's setting your partner's teeth on edge, holding the intention of helping her with her particular issues sets the stage for a meaningful exchange of energy between you.

This is quite different from the type of energy you'll establish if your intention is to slowly arouse your partner with massage for an evening of lovemaking. Your intention needs to be a response to what the recipient of the massage wants and needs, not a tool of manipulation for your own agenda. The more you use intention to consciously meet your romantic partner's expressed needs for stress reduction, pain relief, or whatever her issue truly is, the more likely you are to have her grateful responsiveness after her aches and pains are resolved.

Giving Feedback

When you're receiving massage, you are receiving a gift. And just like your mom had you write thank you notes for gifts you received when you were a kid, it's beneficial to express appreciation for receiving massage, too. The person giving you a massage is taking the time to attend to your comfort, health, and relaxation. Making it clear when something feels good lets him know what you like.

Positive feedback doesn't have to take the form of words. Often "*Mmmmmmmmm*" says it all. If you become nonverbal when you receive massage, valuable feedback in the form of a thumbs-up sign when your massage partner works an area that really needs it or just makes some especially yummy strokes could do the trick. When you're receiving massage in the supine or the side-lying positions where your massage giver can see your face, a broad, relaxed smile tells him when he's doing what you like.

At Your Fingertips

If you're getting a massage and the partner's strokes are too fast, too deep, or otherwise don't suit you, don't just yelp and cringe away from his touch. Instead, try a constructive response such as, "That would feel better if you went a little slower," or "That's an area needs work, but it's a little sore to be worked that deeply." This will get the point across in a positive way.

As you massage, if you get any sense that something you're doing is not comfortable for your partner, ask her about it. You might notice that your partner is getting goose bumps. For some people, this means they're chilly; for others, it means what you're doing feels delicious. The only way to know for sure is to check in. You don't want to keep asking so many questions that your partner can't sink into deep relaxation, but checking in about comfort tells your partner you care about the quality of her massage experience.

The Least You Need to Know

◆ To avoid injury and fatigue when giving a massage, always center, ground, and stretch beforehand to prepare yourself physically as well as mentally.

◆ Communication between the partners during massage is an important part of the experience.

◆ Taking good care of your body and using the right body mechanics enable you to perform good massage without harming yourself.

◆ Proper breathing and energy concerns are very important in providing the best possible massage.

In This Chapter

- ◆ Your bones
- ◆ Your muscles
- ◆ How muscles and bones work together
- ◆ Basic massage strokes

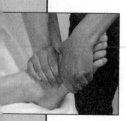
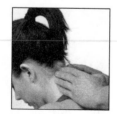
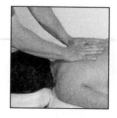
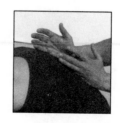
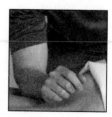
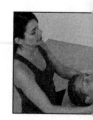

Different Strokes

In Part 2, we give you stroke combinations to use on various areas of the body. Before we get there, though, you need to learn all the strokes you'll use in Part 2's combinations. That's what this chapter is for. We also introduce you to some basic anatomy so you know what you're working on. In preparation for combining the strokes, you learn in this chapter a cohesive massage session. We also orient you to the body with some basic anatomy.

All the strokes can be applied in different ways to different parts of the body. Some are more appropriate for large areas like the back or the thighs. Others are more useful for small areas, like the hands and feet, or around a particular joint. When you know the basics, you'll be able to apply the strokes in creative ways to different areas of the body.

Basic Anatomy

You don't need to be an anatomist to perform a massage, but you do need to know some of the basic terminology to understand what we talk about in later chapters.

When you move, your muscles and bones work together. Muscles connect to bones and move them by pulling on them. Muscles cannot push; they can only pull, so an opposing muscle has to work to move any body part the other way. For example, when you hold your arm down to your side and lift your forearm, your biceps (along with some secondary muscles) contract, pulling on your forearm just forward of your elbow joint. This lifts your forearm. When you lower your forearm back down, part of that movement is accomplished by gravity, but most of the force that moves your forearm down comes from the triceps muscle in the back of your upper arm, contracting and pulling on the back end of your radius bone just back of the elbow joint.

Definition

There's nothing mysterious or even very complicated about basic **anatomy**; it's simply the study of physical structure, in this case the human body. Most people can produce a fairly extensive list of the parts of their cars, with some understanding of what those parts do; surely it's just as interesting to have a clear understanding of our own parts.

Many of the muscles that move parts of your skeleton are located well beyond the bones they move. In this case, you were moving your forearm, but the muscles that facilitate that movement are in your upper arm, with a *tendon* attaching them to the bones in your forearm. Then what do the muscles in your forearm do? Well, they move your hand and fingers. Muscles on the underside of your forearm have long tendons that connect to the bones in your hand and fingers and run out to the tips of your fingers.

Press Here

When we speak of muscles, we are referring to skeletal muscles, or the muscles that act by contracting and applying leverage to move one bone with respect to others. These are the muscles that make voluntary actions, those that we use to make whatever movements we decide to make.

The tendons that connect to the muscles that move your fingers all run through a narrow gap between your wrist bones on the underside of your wrist. This narrow gap surrounding the

tendons is known as the carpal tunnel. We've all heard of carpal tunnel syndrome, a painful inflammation of this area usually caused by prolonged repetitive motion, like typing. (We talk about dealing with carpal tunnel problems in Chapter 18.)

Remembering this indirect connection between muscles and the bones they move can help you understand why painful muscles might not directly relate to the work that made them painful. For example, painful forearm muscles can be the result of doing a lot of work with your fingers. It also explains why massages that are most effective in relieving discomfort in muscles usually are full-body massages.

Frequently, pain is caused by tightness in an area somewhat distant from the area where discomfort is felt. It's amazing how the interactions between different groups of muscles can create imbalances that can cause pain in areas you'd never think of. Part of this is due to the continuity of the connective tissue in the body. Everything in your body is connected in some way with everything else in your body.

Of course, the connection between muscles and the bones they move is not always indirect but always makes perfect sense from a mechanical point of view, and a connection to the part being moved always exists. For example, when you chew, your lower jaw moves up and down with respect to your upper jaw, which is inflexibly fused to your skull. The main muscle used in chewing is the *masseter*, which connects to the underside of the *zygomatic bone* in the skull and runs right down to connect to your lower jaw. You contract this muscle forcefully when you chew, and it's used so frequently that it might contribute to TMJ dysfunction, a painful condition in the tempomandibular joint. (See Chapter 14 for more on TMJ problems.)

The following illustrations provide some useful landmarks on the body, both bones and muscles, so that you'll have a clear idea of what we're referring to in the massage sequences. Having a closer acquaintance with your "parts" can be useful and interesting.

At Your Fingertips

Many of the painful conditions that develop as we age originate in muscular imbalances that pull the bones into misalignment. When bones are not aligned correctly, wear and tear on the joints and joint capsules can result. This sets the stage for arthritic changes in the joints and other conditions like bursitis. Massage can help restore balance between the muscles and prevent or reduce joint damage and dysfunction.

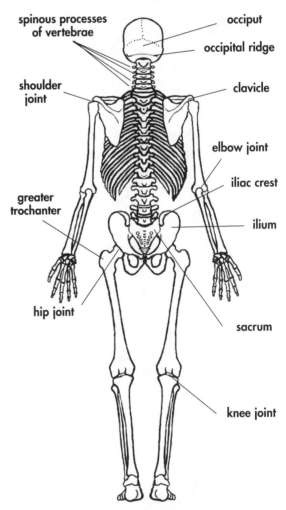

A front view of the human skeleton with the major bones labeled.

A front view of the human skeleton with the major bones labeled.

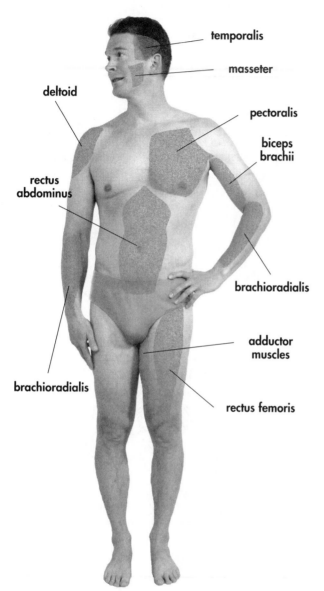

A front view of the body with the major muscles labeled.

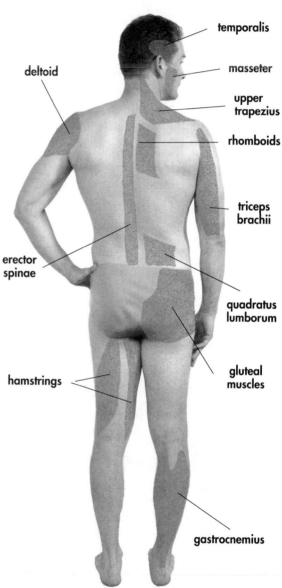

A back view of the body with the major muscles labeled.

The Strokes

Think of this chapter as teaching the letters of the alphabet, and the chapters in Parts 2 and 3 as teaching how to combine those letters into words and phrases. Each individual stroke works with every other stroke to form a complete massage, just as words work together to tell a story. Learning to apply the strokes in the best combinations, becoming literate in the language of massage, is what learning massage is all about.

It's difficult to convey the subtleties of the strokes in still photographs, so we recommend that you view the "Strokes" section of the accompanying DVD for extra instruction.

Effleurage

The first basic stroke is called effleurage. Effleurage is a soothing, flowing stroke used to "open" the area to be worked, whether a limb, the torso, or smaller areas, like the neck and shoulders. Effleurage strokes allow the giver to begin to feel where there might be tension or bound-up areas in the receiver's muscles. Effleurage is useful for spreading the lubricant and making connection with the whole part of the body to be worked on. It's also the stroke for "pulling it all together" after massaging specific areas.

To perform effleurage strokes, lay your hands on the receiver's body with your fingers together and your thumbs parallel to your fingers.

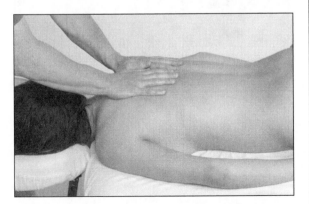

The beginning of an effleurage stroke on the back.

Begin your strokes without pressure and gradually add just a little pressure. Your hands should be molded to the receiver's body in a relaxed, soft way.

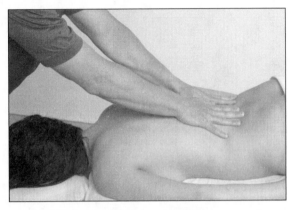

The effleurage stroke is a smooth, flowing stroke applied without a lot of pressure.

Gliding

Gliding is effleurage, but while effleurage is always done with your hands, gliding can also be done with your forearms. Forearm glides can be done on a large area, arm following hand, with pressure exerted from the fingertips all the way to just below the elbow.

Using the "meaty" part of the underside of your forearm or the same part of your forearm, make the stroke a broad one with your forearm perpendicular to the direction of the stroke.

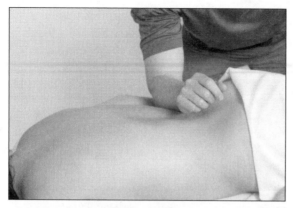

Gliding is modified effleurage that you can do with your forearm.

Petrissage

Petrissage is kneading, a lifting and squeezing of muscles that offers the therapeutic effect of "milking" out the impurities and waste products, which encourages greater circulation and general softening of the muscles. Increased circulation brings more oxygen and nutrients to the cells.

Use your whole hand when applying petrissage, with your fingers together and your thumbs on the other side of the muscle you're working on, keeping your palm in full contact with the muscle.

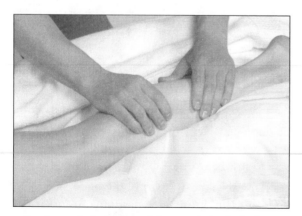

Petrissage is kneading of the muscles to help them loosen up and release tension. It also increases circulation in an area, helping remove waste products and enhance nutrition for the cells.

It's easiest to do on areas such as the neck, arms, and legs, but petrissage can be applied on most areas of the body. The challenge on the back is to keep your entire palm in contact with the muscles while performing the stroke.

Tapotement

Tapotement is French for "tapping," and unlike effleurage and petrissage, it is not an especially relaxing stroke. It can feel invigorating, and it revs up the circulation. Your wrists should be loose when you perform tapotement, both because it feels better to the receiver, and because it is less stressful on your wrists. You should avoid tapotement over the kidney area and on any bony areas. Tapotement is a nice stroke to use toward the very end of a massage session, when it's likely to wake up a sleeping receiver.

There are five types of tapotement:

◆ Hacking is a rhythmic striking using the sides of the hands.

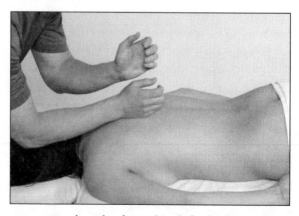

Use the side of your hands for hacking.

At Your Fingertips

It's important to keep your wrists limp and relaxed when performing tapotement, both for the comfort of the receiver and for the health of your wrists.

◆ Beating uses a loose fist.

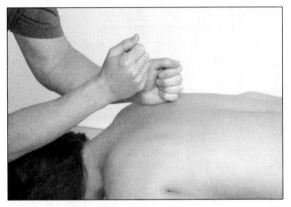

Use a loose fist for beating.

◆ Tapping is tapotement using only the fingertips.

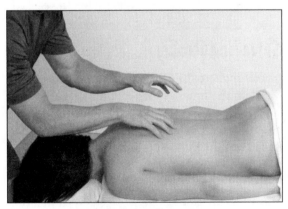

Tap with your fingertips.

◆ Cupping is just what it sounds like—a percussive stroke using the hand in a cupped shape with the fingers together.

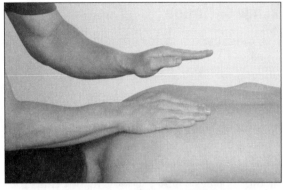

Cupping uses the cupped hand and makes a resonant sound when done properly.

◆ Raindrop tapotement is a specific form of tapping in which the fingers tap in succession, rather than all at once. Raindrop tapotement is generally done on the face.

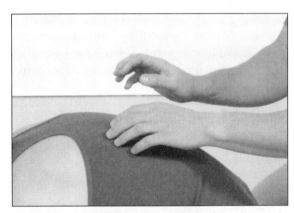

Raindrop tapotement is done with the fingertips and is most commonly done on the face, but can be done on other parts of the body.

Back Off

When doing tapotement on the back, be careful to avoid the area of the kidneys. The kidneys lie on either side of the spine, just above the iliac crest and just below the bottom rib, and extend about 4 inches out from the spine. The kidneys are very sensitive and must be protected from strong percussive blows.

Range of Motion

Per Ling, the originator of Swedish massage, considered movement and joint mobilization an integral part of massage. He called it Swedish gymnastics, which brings to mind a picture that, for most of us, has nothing to do with the actual application of joint mobilization.

Stretching techniques have to be applied carefully, paying attention to the "end points," or those places where the movement begins to come up against resistance. It can be used at any point in the massage session and is often used to loosen up areas that lack normal range of motion.

Examples of range of motion include rocking your partner's torso or legs in either the supine or prone positions, You can rock one bent leg across the other outstretched leg in the supine position. "Sweeping the floor" with the arm, while holding your partner's hand can be useful in helping them release any holding of the arm you are massaging in the supine position. In the side-lying position it is easy to rotate the shoulder through its entire range of motion.

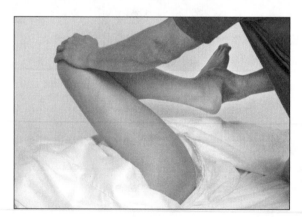

Leg-over stretch and rotation.

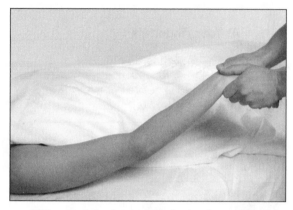

Wrist rotation, shown with the receiver supine.

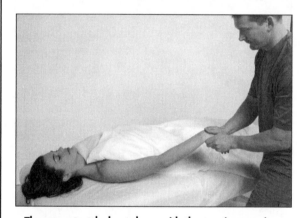

The arm stretch, best done with the receiver supine.

Spreading Strokes

Spreading strokes spread and push downward on the muscles to create more space in an area of the body. The hands start together then move apart, not so much gliding over the surface of the skin as stretching the skin and underlying muscles.

When applied to the forehead, for instance, spreading strokes can help relax and stretch out the contracted tension that results in vertical concentration lines in the middle of the forehead.

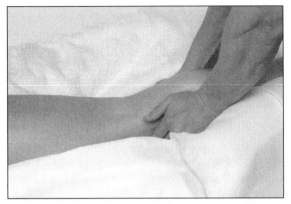

Spreading strokes spread and create more space.

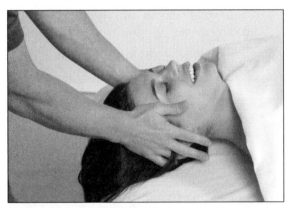

Spreading on the forehead can ease tension lines.

Used on the chest, spreading strokes lengthen the pectoral muscles, which may be shortened due to poor posture, and they enable the shoulders to move back into a more optimal position.

Pin and Stretch

Pin and stretch strokes are modified spreading strokes in which one hand holds or pins a part of the body in place while the other hand spreads and stretches muscles away from the pinned area.

Forearm Rolling

Forearm rolling is a nice way to give your hands a break and is a very full-feeling broadening.

When you're doing this stroke, you roll your forearm so your skin doesn't slide against the receiver's skin.

Start with the underside of your arm resting on the area where you'll perform the rolling action. Lean your weight on your forearm, and rotate your arm so your palm is facing upward. Then you place your arm at the same starting point or another point nearby and repeat the move until you have rolled the entire area.

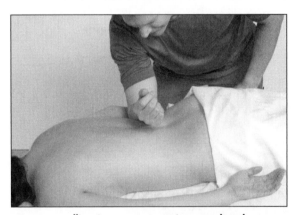

Forearm rolling is one way to give your hands a rest and still continue with effective massage.

Circular and Longitudinal Friction

Circular and straight-line friction can be applied in a number of different ways. One way is to move your hands and forearms in opposite directions, with enough force to move the skin and underlying muscles. Straight-line friction is used mostly on the back. Circular friction performed with the fingertips is useful where muscles attach to bones, such as around the edges of the scapula, and is used on many different areas of the body.

Circular friction is most commonly applied with just the fingers or thumbs. Circular friction used near the joints has an effect on the entire muscle or muscles that have attachments at that point. Often, when you apply friction near a joint, you'll feel ropey bands of tissue where the tendons are tight. Friction is also a very good tool for palpation.

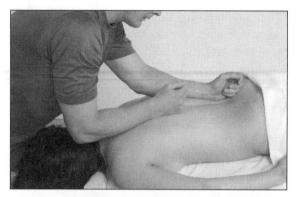

Longitudinal friction used on the back creates heat and loosens the back muscles.

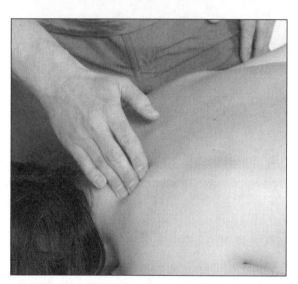

Friction around the scapula is useful for both palpation and for relaxing the attached muscles.

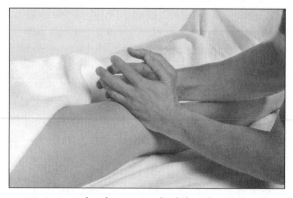

Friction can be done using both hands moving in opposite directions.

Vibration

Like a rock thrown into a still pool, the ripples from vibration oscillate out into muscles some distance from the point where you apply the vibration. Vibration is of two sorts:

◆ Fine vibration is a very small, rapid vibrating of your fingers that comes all the way from your shoulder and is applied to a small area, from which it radiates out into a small area of the body.

◆ Coarse vibration is rocking and rolling a whole area of the body and can be very comforting. You can use coarse vibration to increase the range of motion of joints, and to confuse muscles into letting go and relaxing.

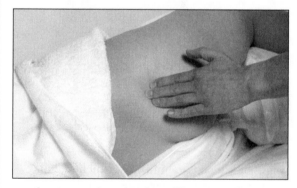

Vibration can have rippling effects some distance away from where you apply it.

Wringing

Wringing, a variation of which is sometimes called "ocean waves" when applied over a broad area, uses the hands passing each other as they move in opposite directions. The politically incorrect "Indian burn" or "Indian rub" Wringing feels really good when the skin is well lubricated. It is often used on the feet and ankles as well as the wrists and forearms.

Press Here

Palpation is the evaluation of muscle through sensitive use of the hands. By palpating, you feel for any areas of a muscle that feel different—dense, ropey, congested, tight, or with trigger points that may feel like anything from a pea to a golf ball. It's important to maintain focus while you're palpating muscle tissue. You might want to close your eyes to eliminate the distraction of sight and avoid conversation with the receiver while you're feeling tissue quality, except to ask about whether an area you have located is painful. (For more on palpation, see Chapter 16.)

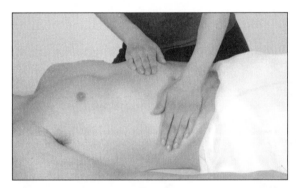

Wringing can be used on wrists, ankles, or on larger areas, as "ocean waves."

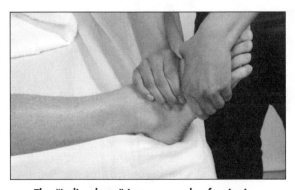

The "Indian burn" is an example of wringing.

Raking

Raking is a pulling and lifting stroke that uses the fingers rather than the palm of the hand. This vigorous stroke lifts and firms the skin and underlying muscles. It can also be helpful in relaxing a muscle that's gone into spasm.

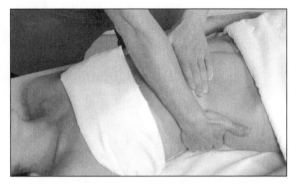

Raking uses pulling strokes on the abdomen. Note you can reach around to the receiver's side for a longer pull.

The Least You Need to Know

◆ Bones and other connective tissue form the support for everything else in the body. Muscles move bones.

◆ Learning a little about anatomy helps you give better massages.

◆ Massages are built from a small number of basic strokes. Learn the strokes, and you're partway there.

In This Part

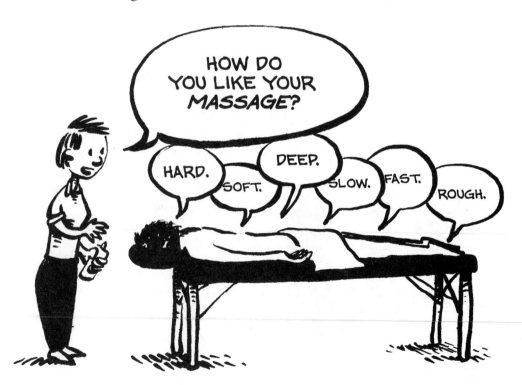

Part 2

Combining Strokes

In Part 2, we take the basic stroke techniques you learned in Chapter 2 and show you how to combine them and apply them to specific areas of the body. If you think of Part 1 as learning the alphabet, Part 2 is learning to combine those letters into words, phrases, and sentences. Each area of the body you're massaging needs its own individually crafted sentence. What's right for the neck is not right for the abdomen; the back has different needs than the hips; and so on. Read the chapters in Part 2, practice the sequences for each part of the body, and soon you will be performing massages that completely relax and sooth your partner.

In This Chapter

- ◆ The importance of head and face massage
- ◆ Preparation and first touch
- ◆ The right strokes for the head and face
- ◆ Tips on using care and sensitivity when massaging

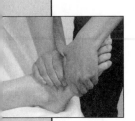
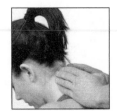
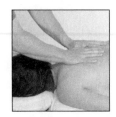
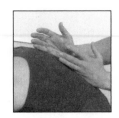
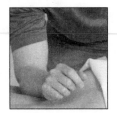
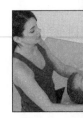

Chapter 5

The Head and Face

The head and face are very important areas in massage. If you can relax a person's head and face (and neck, covered more in Chapters 6 and 7), you're on the right track toward relaxing the entire person.

Massaging these potentially sensitive areas isn't as simple as it might seem, however. The head houses the delicate balance mechanisms of the inner ears. In addition, an especially large number of sensory nerves are located in the head and face area, second only to the hands. Many people are very touchy around their eyes, so work slowly, gently, and conservatively here.

Be sure you are relaxed before you work on someone else, or you'll transmit the tension you're holding in your upper body and arms to your partner. It's very important that you be centered, grounded, and relaxed before you begin massaging a person's head area. Every movement you make on a person's head is magnified and feels five times as fast and five times as large to him. Always keep this in mind, and go slowly and gently when working on this area.

A Few Notes Before You Start

A good facial or head massage can feel heavenly. Before you put your hands on someone else, though, let's go over a few massage tips.

If you're using a lotion, work it into your hands well before starting to massage the face. Use light lotion rather than a rich cream on facial areas; often you don't even need much lubricant for the face, as it tends to have more natural oil than other areas of the body.

At Your Fingertips

If you feel tense, go back through the centering and grounding exercises in Chapter 3 before massaging anyone.

For people who are prone to acne, it might be best to not use any potentially pore-clogging lubricants. Depending on the severity of the acne, it might be best for you to only do a few feathery strokes on the face. Be careful to avoid any deeper work that could be painful, irritate the acne bumps, or spread infection.

Back Off

A person with acne might be sensitive or embarrassed about the condition and prefer that you avoid massaging his face. One way to deal with this sensitive issue is to ask if he would like you to massage his face without mentioning the acne.

Remember, too, that many people prefer not to get lotion, oil, or cream in their hair. If you've lubricated your hands for previous parts of the massage, wipe off any excess oil or lotion before massaging the scalp.

Be aware that gravity is doing an adequate job, thank you very much, of dragging down the facial muscles and skin, so avoid adding to gravity's effect by pulling the facial skin downward. Your strokes should be encouraging, upward, and outward. Most of us contract our facial muscles toward the center of our faces when we're unhappy, angry, or concentrating, so smoothing works best if it's done from the center toward the ears. No fish faces, please!

First Touch: The Forehead

To give a head massage, start at front and center: the forehead. Have the receiver lie supine (face up) on a massage table or on the floor, with a pillow or other bolster under his lower thigh and knee area to avoid aggravating any possible lower back strain. Be sure he is warm and comfortable.

Sit comfortably on a chair or stool (or cross-legged on the floor at his head) at a height that allows your shoulders to be in a relaxed and neutral position while you work on the receiver's face and head. This goes a long way toward ensuring that you're not holding tension and transferring it to your receiver.

1. Start with a contact hold, slowly lowering your thumbs to his forehead, with the inner edges of your thumbs together.

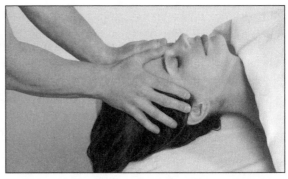

Begin each portion of a massage with a contact hold on the area of the body you'll be massaging.

2. Rest your hands gently on his head for three to five of his breaths.

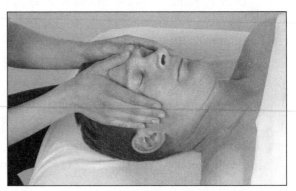

Let your hands rest on his head for a few breaths.

3. Stroke out from the center of his forehead toward his ears.

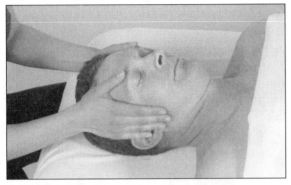

Glide outward from his forehead.

4. Lean forward, applying gentle pressure on his forehead, and slowly allow your thumbs to slide out all the way to the front margin of his ears.

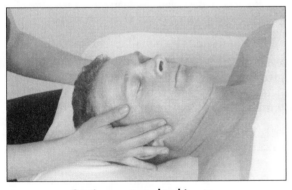

Continue outward to his ears.

5. Repeat two or three times.

Back Off _____

Take extra care to avoid bumping his ears throughout the massage. That's one of the quickest ways of destroying relaxation, and is right up there with working too close to the eyes.

This stroke starts to iron out the vertical tension lines in the forehead that often come from concentration, squinting, and emotional disturbance.

Temple Circles

After the forehead stroke, move your hands out toward his ears and begin to make friction circles on his temples with your fingers. Use the pads on your fingertips, and be sure to make the circles large enough to go up into the hairline above his ears. Make at least 8 to 12 circles before moving on.

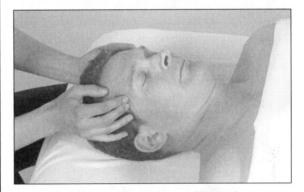

Perform circular friction on the temples.

Anytime you work on the scalp, apply firm pressure, enough to move the scalp and not just move over the hair, which makes annoying "scratchy noises" that could distract your receiver.

Gliding on the Side of the Face

After the temple circles, begin working from under his chin to the top of his head:

1. Place your hands gently under his chin.

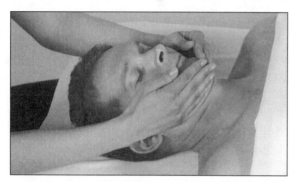

Start with both hands under his chin.

2. Glide the fingers of each hand up the sides of his face, over his temples, and all the way to the top of his head.

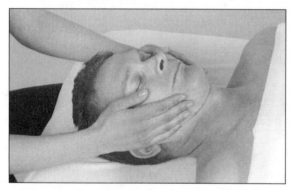

Use smooth, gliding strokes upward on his face.

3. Notice how his facial muscles take on the look of a smile as you do this stroke, which can only be good.

4. Repeat two to five times.

Back Off _____

Be particularly careful when working around the eyes if your receiver wears contact lenses or has had any eye surgery.

Scalp Circles

After your last upward gliding stroke, and with your hands at the top of his head, begin to apply circular friction strokes on his scalp. Again, use your fingers with enough pressure that you're actually moving his scalp rather than just moving over his hair.

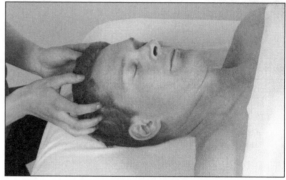

Use your fingers when making scalp circles with enough pressure to move the scalp.

As you make these small circles all over his scalp, be alert for areas that feel tighter, and give them special attention. You could also clasp hanks of his hair right at the scalp and pull lightly as you make circles. This is great for loosening a tight scalp, where many people tend to carry tension.

Back Off _____

Before doing any sort of scalp massage, be sure you know if your receiver has had hair implants or weaves. If he's had this kind of augmentation, it's best to avoid scalp massage rather than take a risk on displacing anything.

Say What? The Ears

Next, you're going to focus on his ears. Having your ears rubbed in this way feels great!

1. Begin with your fingers spread on each side of his ears, and work with a gentle upward stroke. We call this stroke the "Why dogs think we're gods" stroke.

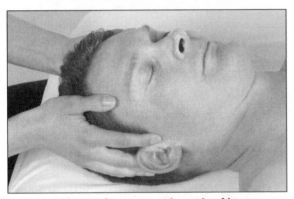

Start with your fingers on either side of his ears.

2. As your hands move from his scalp back down to his ears, spread your fingers far enough apart so your index fingers are just forward of his ears and your middle fingers are behind them.

3. Move your fingers up and down at the edge of his face and behind his ears, using more pressure as your fingers pull back up toward his temples, and lighter pressure when your fingers move down toward his jaw.

4. Repeat five to eight times.

More Ears: Going in Circles

If he doesn't have a prohibitive number of ear piercings, make small circles with your thumbs and index fingers on each side of his ear lobes.

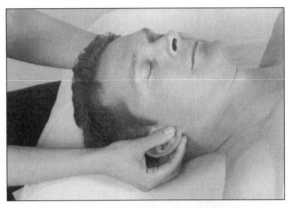

Continue to the earlobes.

Next, work up and around his *ear pinnae*.

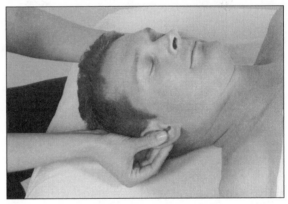

Now work on the outer part of the ear.

Definition

The **pinna** (plural: *pinnae*) is the outer portion of the ear. It's often what we think of when we think of ears because it's the part we can see.

This massage feels delightful to most people. In addition, numerous reflexology points are located around the ear. This massage might stimulate them in the process. (For more on reflexology, see Chapter 17.)

Jaws: Relieving Tension

Many people carry tension in their jaws. This is a classic place to store anger and undelivered communication, which builds until jaw muscles tighten and cause all sorts of problems. But jaw tension can also result from misaligned teeth, holding a pipe between the teeth, dental procedures, or chewing gum.

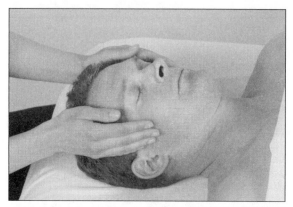

Relaxing the jaw goes a long way toward relaxing the whole person.

At Your Fingertips

It's a good idea to ask the receiver to get rid of any chewing gum before a massage session. It's almost impossible for him to really relax when his jaw is busy chewing. Best for the giver not to chew gum either, as it can be very distracting for the person receiving the massage.

Begin with circular strokes similar to those you used on his temples, and progress down his jaw using short, downward strokes with moderate pressure. Press hard enough to reach the muscles that move the jaw. Repeat for 10 to 20 jaw circles.

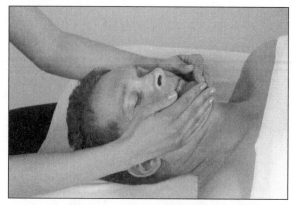

Work on the jaw with circular strokes as well as short, downward strokes.

You could also use a stroke here called the "pinch." Use your fingers and thumbs to gently pinch the edge of his jaw, moving your hands from the middle of his chin along the edge of his jaw up to just below his ear. Do one or two pinches along his jaw line before moving on.

If you're uncertain exactly where the jaw muscles are (the muscles used in chewing and that tend to hold tension), put your hand on the receiver's jaw area and ask him to clench his back teeth briefly. Where you feel a hard knot form is the muscle you want to work on.

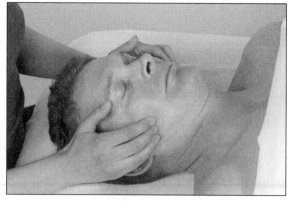

Be careful in the lower cheek area if your receiver has any kind of dental work.

After he's relaxed his jaw again, use circular friction to address these hard-working and very strong facial muscles. This is also the only place on the face you'll want to make deep downward strokes. Small, short, relatively deep "stripping" or one-way strokes from below his cheekbone down to his jaw line help ease the tension held in this area. Repeat 10 to 20 times.

At Your Fingertips

Be very careful when doing deep work on the lower cheeks if the receiver has orthodontic braces or wears dentures.

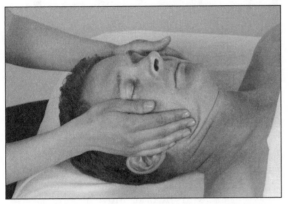

These very short strokes from the cheekbone to the jaw are the only time you'll use downward pressure on the face.

If he can't loosen his jaw tension, you might want to ask him to place the edge of his tongue between his back teeth to make your stroke more effective. This helps keep him from clenching his teeth and "fighting" the stroke. Or he could just allow his mouth to hang open, but many people are resistant to doing that.

Back Off

Never try to force anyone's jaw to relax. If he grinds his teeth at night or clenches them during the day (or both), he might be unable to release the tension in his jaw muscles. It might only irritate him if you keep trying to release that tension.

Outward Strokes Below the Cheekbones

Continuing on this massage journey, next comes the cheekbones:

1. Bring your index and middle finger pads to the base of his nasal bones, right at the top of the crease by the sides of his nose.

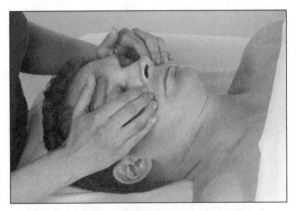

Begin the cheekbone stroke at the crease beside his nose.

2. Make a few firm effleurage strokes from the edges of his nose, right below the cheekbones, all the way out to the point where the top of his ear joins his face.

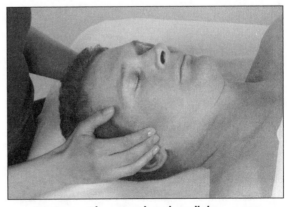

Continue with outward strokes all the way to his ears.

3. There's a small indentation at this spot, which is a useful acupressure point for headaches. You might feel a slight pulse under your fingertips at this point. Pause here in front of his ear before you repeat the stroke.

4. Repeat two to four times.

The Neck

The neck is another common place people hold tension and stress, so we bet you won't find many people who turn down your offer of a neck massage!

When working on the neck, it's best to begin with alternating hand-pulling strokes:

1. Bring one hand, palm up, under his neck as close to his shoulders as you can reach. Keeping full contact with the entire back of his neck, slide your hand all the way up his neck and a few inches up the back of his head in a firm effleurage pulling stroke. Don't lift up his head as you bring your hand toward your chest, but allow your hand to slide along the sheet under his head.

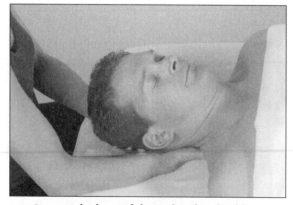

Start on the base of the neck at his shoulders.

2. As soon as your first hand gets to the back of his head, start the same pulling stroke on the back of his neck with your other hand.

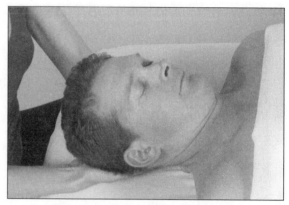

Use pulling strokes up the back of the neck and head.

3. Repeat this stroke six to eight times initially and in between working on other parts of the head, face, and neck. This is one stroke no one seems to be able to get too much of!

Don't allow his head to move around as you pull. It helps to lean back so you increase your stability. He'll feel that his head is being securely and solidly supported. If you let his head move around a lot as you do this stroke, he'll try to hold his head up for you, which is not relaxing for him at all.

If you're not "bobbling" his head and he still can't seem to relax his head and neck tension, you might want to ask him to allow his head to be heavy. You might also suggest that he focus on breathing deeply into his belly. Sometimes the harder someone tries to relax, the harder it is to do!

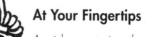 **At Your Fingertips**

Avoid massaging the front of the neck. Most people are not comfortable with someone's hands in this vulnerable area.

Loosening the Long Neck Muscles

Continue with circular friction on the back of his neck. With your palms still facing upward and the backs of your hands resting on the sheet, make small mirror-image circles on the pronounced muscles on each side of his spine. You can make these circles with your fingers as you move gradually up and down the back of his neck and then back and forth across the base of his skull, where a lot of tension-holding muscles are located. Continue with the circles for about 3 minutes; the number of circles would not be less than 60.

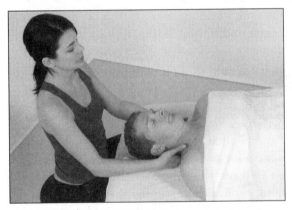

Continue with circular friction on each side of the spine.

![hand icon] **Back Off** _____

Strictly avoid putting pressure on the spinous processes of the vertebrae. These are the protruding bumps of the spine you can feel along his backbone and on the back of his neck.

More Neck: On the Side

After working the back of his neck, it's time to move to the sides:

1. Slowly and gently bring his head to the left, keeping your left hand under the base of his skull behind his left ear to maintain the side stretch to the left on his neck.

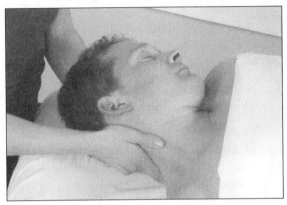

Gently move his head to one side.

2. It might be helpful to move a little to the left side as you're tilting his head in that direction. This will make it easier for your right hand to go from his neck just below and behind his ear, right down his neck, around his right shoulder from front to back, and then return up his neck from behind.

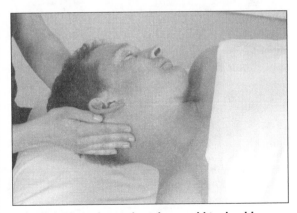

Glide down his neck and around his shoulder.

3. Do this flowing effleurage stroke four to six times before moving his head to the other side and repeating.

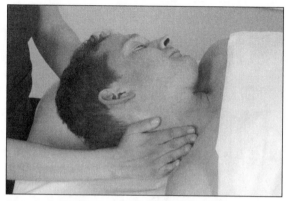

Continue with flowing effleurage.

It's nice to do a few more pulling strokes on his neck, massaging both sides together, before you do a contact hold on the sides of his face or on his shoulders and move on to other parts of body.

If at any point while you're massaging a body area your hand wants to slow down or stop, you're probably sensing an increased density in the tissue. This comes from tension held in the muscles. Hang out on these areas, allowing the warmth and pressure of your hand to encourage the muscle tension to "melt."

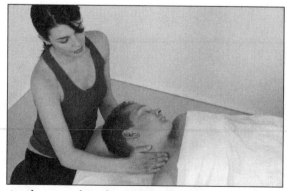

Let the warmth and pressure of your hand melt away his tension.

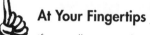 **At Your Fingertips**

If you allow your hand to stop on and compress a tense area and feel a pulse there, move your hand slightly until you no longer feel the pulse. You don't want to interrupt the flow of blood to his brain!

A Few Closing Thoughts

When working on the neck, always start your strokes lightly and only gradually increase the pressure, watching his face for any sign of a grimace. Also watch for other signs of discomfort such as clenched fists, trying to move away from your hands, or jumping. (Fortunately, most of the time when he jumps, it'll be because he's begun to drift off to sleep, which means you're doing your job well and he's relaxing!)

It's helpful to ask if your pressure level is okay if you detect any signs of discomfort. We often have the tendency to give the kind of massage we would personally like to receive. Particularly if you like very deep massage, you must resist the temptation to work too deeply on your receiver, who may not like really deep massage. Always remember that it's his session, not yours, and his preferences are what matter.

The Least You Need to Know

◆ The head, face, and neck are among the most important areas to concentrate on during a massage.

◆ It is easiest to massage the head, face, and neck if the receiver is lying supine (face up) on a massage table, but it can also be done on the floor with a mat.

◆ Ears are important in head massage because they are sensitive and harbor reflexology points.

◆ Always start your massage in this area with gentle strokes and get a feel for how much pressure feels right to your receiver.

In This Chapter

- ◆ A quick and relaxing massage when you don't have a lot of time

- ◆ Help relieve pent-up upper body stress with massage moves that are easy on the giver

- ◆ Simple massage-area setup not requiring special equipment tips

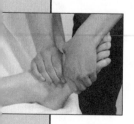
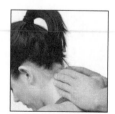
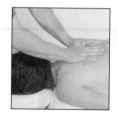
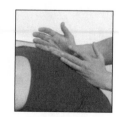
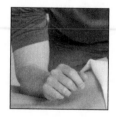
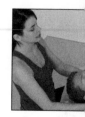

Chapter 6

The Neck, Shoulders, and Upper Back–Seated

Many of the stresses that keep us from being able to take time for a relaxing full-body massage are the same stresses that lodge as tension in our necks, shoulders, and upper backs. The time we spend sitting at desks and computers, sitting or standing while working on assembly lines, and commuting in stop-and-go traffic all contribute to tension and pain that not only affect the neck, shoulders, and upper back, but can radiate into the arms and hands, or even up into the head. Releasing as much of this tension as possible can improve quality of life and performance on and off the job.

Massage-Area Setup

Very little setup is required for a relaxing and renewing upper body massage session, and it can be done almost anywhere. Find a narrow chair without arms or a stool that's the right height to allow the receiver's feet to rest firmly on the floor. Place the back of the chair against a table if one is available. Place two or three large pillows on the table and another pillow in the chair, propped up against the back of the chair. Having another chair or stool for you to sit on allows you to work without hyper-extending your wrists.

Have the receiver straddle the chair. Adjust the pillow in front of his torso and the ones piled in front of him so he can comfortably lean into the pillows.

Back Off

When the back of your hand is close to 90 degrees (perpendicular) to your arm this is considered hyper-extension. In itself it may not be a hazard to your wrist health, but if you apply pressure with your wrist in this position, especially if you do so repeatedly, you possibly can create pain and injury.

If you want to go further, you might want to check out a massage chair. These have the advantage of greater adjustability and offer your partner more precision of support. See Appendix A for more information on massage chairs.

Hands On!

This seated chair-massage sequence is adapted in part from a Thai yoga massage form usually performed on a floor mat. (You can do it that way if you prefer.) It requires that the receiver sit comfortably in a cross-legged position while you're massaging him and that you have the flexibility to kneel, sit on your heels, and keep your balance in those positions.

At Your Fingertips

If necessary, your partner can hold a pillow or two in his lap. He can use these for support if he needs to bend forward more than he would in the seated chair massage.

1. Stand behind your partner and get grounded and centered.

2. Place your hands on his shoulders for a contact hold. Hold this for several of his breaths.

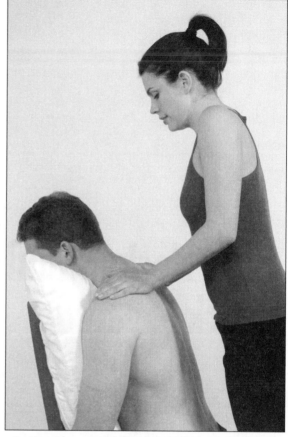

Begin with contact hold on the receiver's shoulders.

Circles on the Back of the Neck

Now it's time to really get to work. These back-of-the-neck circles will really release tension.

1. After a few breaths, place your hands on the back of his neck and get in touch with his neck muscles first with some effleurage, palpating for areas of dense, tight muscle, or ropey bands.

2. As you begin to explore the tissue more deeply, begin to apply circular friction on each side of the spine with your fingers, moving up and down the taut bands of muscle. When you happen upon a place

that feels especially tight or congested, allow your fingers to remain in contact with the area with moderate pressure. Usually the tension begins to melt after 30 seconds or so.

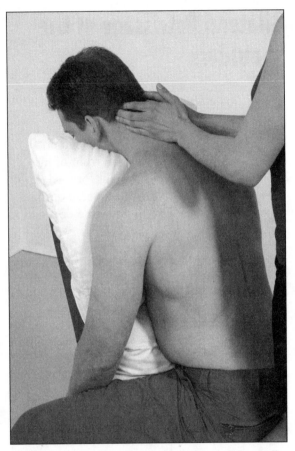

Move on to applying friction to the base of the skull.

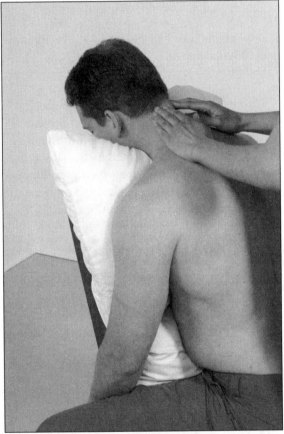

Use your fingers to apply circular friction to the back of the receiver's neck.

3. After three or four sets of circles up and down his neck, come to the base of his skull and continue the circular friction back and forth across his *occiput*.

Definition

The base of the skull at the back is called the **occiput**. It is an important area in head and neck massage because most of the neck muscles, and some of the shoulder muscles have attachments on this bony area.

4. Close by smoothing over with a little more effleurage, stroking down his neck and around his shoulders a minimum of three or four times.

Bilateral Petrissage of the Shoulders

Along with the neck, the shoulders are a key area many people hold stress and tension. Petrissage will really loosen the area.

With your hands on his upper shoulders, begin by bracing your fingers in front of his shoulders and bring your thumbs forward toward your fingers. This will squeeze out tension from this area. Do this at least a dozen times.

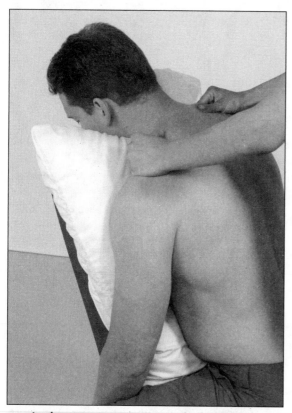

Apply squeezing petrissage to both shoulders.

Back Off

Stay clear of the spinous processes of the vertebrae on the neck and upper back as you perform this work. They are delicate structures, and not only will it be uncomfortable for the receiver if you press on them, but if the receiver is fine-boned or has weakened bone structure, you could actually damage the bone.

Alternately, you can brace your thumbs and the heel of your hand on the back of his shoulder and bring your fingers back toward your thumbs, squeezing as directed earlier. It's a good idea to check in to see which variation the receiver prefers—you never know if you don't ask (unless he volunteers the information).

Palming the Shoulders

More shoulder work. For this part of the massage, stand behind your partner as he sits upright rather than leaning into the pillows.

At Your Fingertips

If you have trouble leaning your weight into the following strokes, or if you're raising up your shoulders to perform them, find either a shorter chair for your partner to sit on, or something sturdy for you to stand on that will give you the height to apply downward pressure effectively.

1. Lift and squeeze the shoulder muscles, starting at the base of the neck and gradually working all the way out to the *deltoid muscles*, applying at least 20 petrissage strokes. Be sure to keep your entire palm on the area as you work so it doesn't feel "pinchy" to the receiver.

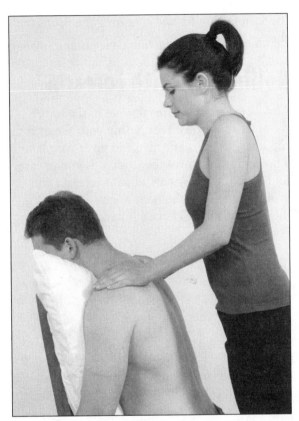

Apply lifting and squeezing pressure with
your palms.

Definition

The main large muscles that cap the
shoulders are known as the **deltoid
muscles,** due to their triangular or
delta shape.

2. As you knead the area, feel for areas of
   tension and lean into them with compression for 30 seconds or so, or until you feel
   the tension begin to melt.

3. Resume the shoulder petrissage. You can
   do a variation of the lifting and squeezing
   movement by keeping your thumbs and
   heels of your hands stationary on the back
   of the his upper shoulder and squeezing

the muscles downward with your fingers moving toward your palms. Imagine
kneading dough.

Alternately, try keeping your fingers stationary on the front of his shoulders, and
compress the muscles with your thumbs
moving toward your fingers. Ask him
which variation he prefers.

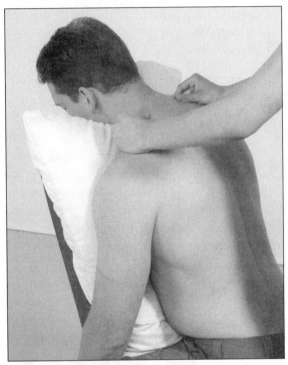

Your receiver might prefer this squeezing motion on
the shoulder muscles.

4. Still standing, lean your palms, fingers facing upward, onto his shoulders with your
   hands close in to his neck.

At Your Fingertips

The downward pressure should come
from leaning onto his shoulders with
your body weight, not from arm pressure.
Find something stable to stand on, if necessary, so you can lean your body weight
into the shoulder muscles.

5. Coordinate your pressure so you're lean-ing onto his shoulders as he exhales and releasing the pressure as he inhales. Do at least six repetitions of this pressure.

Back Off

Avoid using pressure as you go over the clavicle (collarbone) and parts of the scapula (shoulder blade). These bones are close to the surface in the upper shoulder area, and it may cause discomfort for your receiver if you press too vigorously on them.

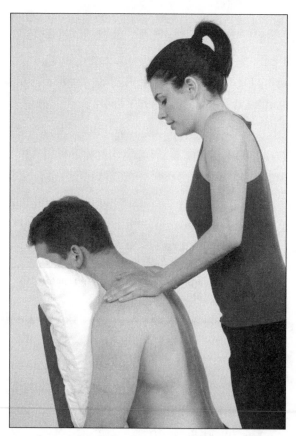

Use the weight of your body to produce the pressure.

You can vary the palming compression by turning your hands so your fingers point out to the sides of his shoulders or by taking your hands a few inches behind and below his upper (trapezius) muscles and repeating the palming there.

Rolling Pin with Forearm

Almost everyone carries tension in the upper shoulder (trapezius) area. Using your forearm to roll out tension is effective and gives your hands a break during a massage session. If you're care-ful to use the fleshy part of your forearm and avoid rolling with the bony areas of your arm, this movement will have a broad, deep feel to your partner.

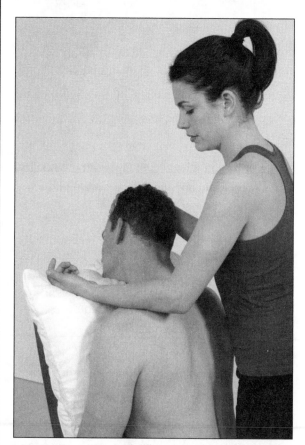

The "rolling pin" motion with your forearm is great for relaxing tension in muscles of the upper shoulder.

1. Working in the same position, use your hands to gently lean the receiver's head to the left, holding it in that position with your left hand.

2. Place the meaty part of your right forearm close to his neck on his trapezius, with your palm facing downward.

3. Roll your forearm so your palm is facing upward, and repeat, each time rolling in the same direction, about a dozen times. Avoid rolling over the bony parts of his shoulder, especially if your arms are thin.

4. Repeat on the other side.

Triceps Rotations and Stretch with Squeeze

The *triceps* muscle on the back of the arm is frequently ignored, but it is, along with the better-known biceps muscle, one of the work horses of the upper arm. Most of us don't notice when the triceps muscle is tired and overworked until it receives nurturing attention in the form of massage. The arm rotations will warm the triceps up for the kneading and stretching that follow. By adding a stretch to this massage movement, you can offer added relief from soreness and tightness in the muscle. Be careful to keep your palm fully on the arm as you apply petrissage; this is an area where a pinching feeling will definitely not be appreciated.

Definition _____

The large muscle on the back of the upper arm is known as the **triceps**.

1. With the receiver still seated in an upright position, reach down and lift up his arm, just using your fingers under his elbow.

2. When you get the upper arm up by the side of his head, take his wrist in your other hand and make slow, sweeping arcs with his arm up, over, and behind his head, always feeling for the end points, or

places where you can feel that it would be a strain to stretch his arm farther.

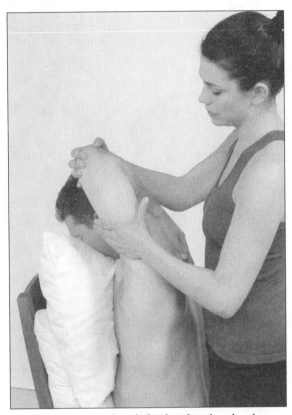

Bring his arm up beside his head and make slow, sweeping arcs with his arm.

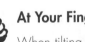 **At Your Fingertips** _____

When tilting the receiver's head to the side or putting his arm or shoulder into a stretch, honor his flexibility limitation. There's a remarkable difference in people's range of motion in joints, and it can be uncomfortable and possibly dangerous to exceed a receiver's normal range.

3. Make 8 to 10 slow circles with his arm to loosen up his shoulder.

4. After the arm circles, place his hand behind his neck, and reach over to pull his elbow in a little closer to his head.

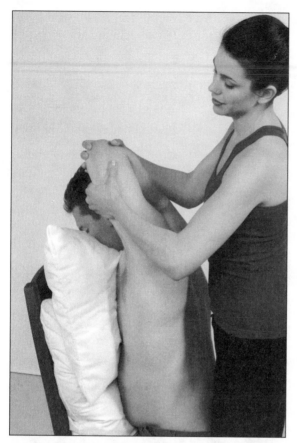

Place his hand behind his neck, and pull his elbow closer to his head.

5. Using your hand closest to his upraised arm, apply petrissage to the triceps muscle from his elbow to near his armpit and back to his elbow.

6. Make three or four more revolutions of his arm before you place the arm back down, again holding his elbow to move his arm.

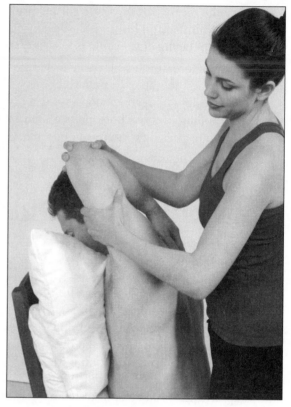

With his elbow in closer to his head, apply petrissage to his triceps muscle.

Neck Massage

Computers, and especially laptop computers, cause us to hold our heads in rigid positions for extended time periods. The resulting tension in our necks can cause pain not just in the neck, but in the head and the shoulders as well. Massaging your partner's neck in the seated position allows you the ease of working with gravity in providing a stretch as you apply effleurage and petrissage to the muscles that support and move the head.

Back Off

Exercise extreme caution when massaging anyone who is under the care of a medical professional for any neck or back injuries, or who is receiving care for any ongoing conditions.

1. Gently lean the receiver's head forward, and lace your fingers together on the back of his neck. Watch your own body mechanics here. Bend at your knees rather than bending over at your lower back to avoid straining your back.

2. With your elbows out to the side at about your chest level and your laced fingers toward you, place the heels of your hands at the side of the receiver's neck.

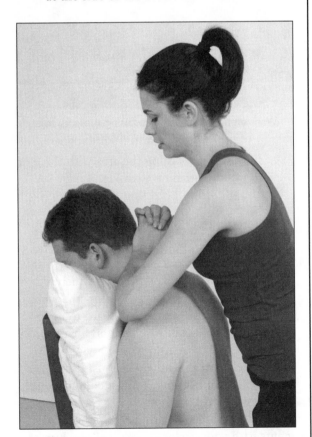

Use the heels of your hands on the sides of his neck.

3. Slowly bring the heels of your hands together, coming off the back of his neck at the end of each stroke.

4. Repeat six or eight times.

Shoulder Massage

When we're cold, stressed, or feel threatened in some way, our shoulders seem to automatically rise up toward our ears. This requires a sustained action of the upper trapezius and other upper shoulder muscles, and they can become fatigued and sore. Massaging your partner's shoulders in the seated position allows you to maintain a neutral position of your own shoulders while easing the tension out of his.

It is estimated that 90 percent of all adults have pain-producing trigger points in their upper shoulder muscles. You can develop the skill to ease this discomfort by using these simple techniques of effleurage, petrissage and friction. Palpation is a technique used to explore what is going on in the muscles, but it is far more than that: as you palpate the muscle attachments to a bone you are releasing tension and discomfort as well.

1. With the receiver leaning forward into the pillows, takes a seat in your chair. You should be sitting fairly close to him so you don't have to lean forward or stretch to get to his shoulders. You might need a pillow in your chair to be at a good height to massage his shoulders without fatiguing your arms.

2. Warm up his back by making six to eight effleurage strokes up and down his whole back, coming around his shoulders.

3. Then settle into exploring the contours of his shoulder blades. You might start at any edge of these triangular bones and work your way around them, alternately using your fingers or thumbs in the various areas

(whichever keeps your wrists in a neutral position).

So many muscles attach to the *scapula*, and by performing friction strokes around the edges of the bone, you are massaging the attachment points for all the muscles in the area. This friction really feels great.

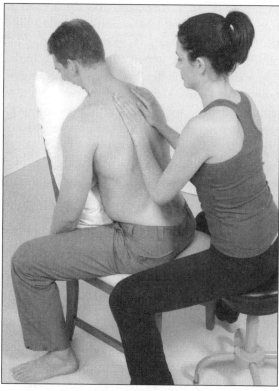

Be sure you're at the right height to easily reach his shoulders without straining or overtiring your arms.

Definition

The large, flattened triangular bone on the back of each shoulder, commonly called the shoulder blade, is technically called the **scapula** (plural *scapulae*). The scapula has muscles attached all around its periphery that provide stability for the upper back and movement of the arm at the shoulder. The bone and the associated muscles make up a very important area for shoulder and back massage.

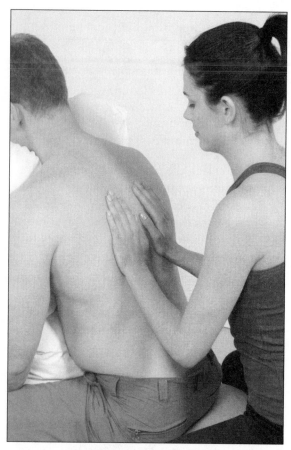

Work on his shoulder blades using pressure from your thumbs and fingers.

4. Finish by smoothing the area with three or four more effleurage strokes.

Back Massage

By performing compression strokes to each side of the vertebral column, what we frequently refer to as the spine, you can address the whole length of the muscles that work hard to maintain our upright posture. It's important to use your arms as extensions of your moving body to create the strokes rather than just using your arms. It feels much more connected to have the compressive strokes coming from the movement of your body. Coordinating your movements with your partner's breath allows him to relax into the strokes and have some feeling that he is controlling the pace of the compressions.

1. With the receiver still leaning into the pillows in front of him, place your palms to each side of his spine on his lower back. Take a seat behind him for this portion of the massage to protect your back.

2. Press in, using your body weight rather than arm strength, in coordination with his exhalations. On his inhalations, release the pressure, slide your hands upward a few inches, and repeat on the next exhalation, gradually walking your hands all the way up to his lower shoulders and then walking them back down to his lower back again. You will press your hands into his back muscles in about six positions on your way up and then again on the way back down his back.

3. From his lower back, reach around to his sides and find the *iliac crest* (more prominent at the side of the body). Explore the crest with circular friction all the way back to his spine, and then continue the circular friction back around to his sides, for about a minute. Numerous muscles attach to the *ilium*, and it feels great when you work them close to the bone.

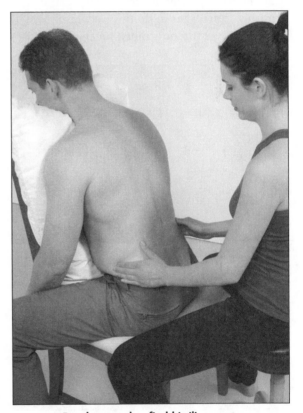

Reach around to find his iliac crest.

Definition

The pelvis is made up of several parts. The two large bones on the sides are the **ilia** (singular *ilium*). The flared upper part of the ilium, which serves as the attachment point for many muscles, is called the **iliac crest,** and may be explored with your fingers.

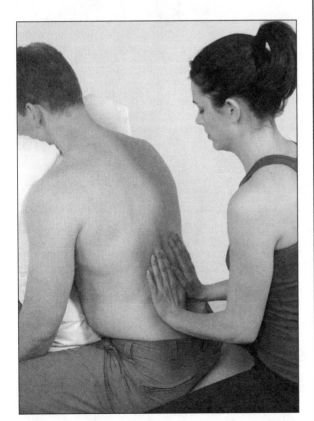

Use your palms to apply pressure to the lower back.

Longitudinal Friction on Each Side of the Spine

With the receiver still leaning forward and supported by the pillows, place your forearms on either side of his spine, with your palms facing each other, and slide your arms vigorously up and down the muscles, creating friction and heat. This is challenging for your body and you probably won't want to do this for more than 30 seconds, no matter how much he enjoys it.

2. Start by rhythmically hacking with the side of your hands up and down his back. Keep your wrists loose and floppy, as it protects them from injury and feels better to the receiver. This is a short sequence, just 20 seconds or so, just long enough to wake your receiver up from the nap you've put him into.

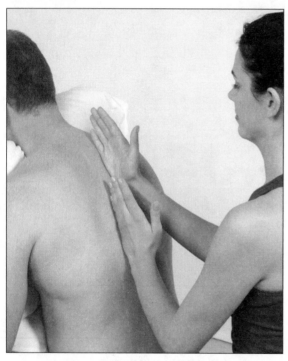

Use your forearms on each side of the spine to create friction and heat.

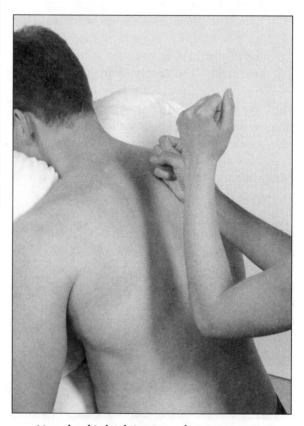

Now that his back is warmed up, move on to tapotement.

Tapotement on Back

Move right into tapotement on his back while it's warmed up.

1. Put one hand on each side of his spine in the same orientation you used for longitudinal friction.

Back Off

Be very cautious about giving massage to anyone who tells you he is taking any medication for pain, as he won't be able to give you valid feedback on how your massage feels to him.

3. Change your hand position by clenching your hands into loose fists, continuing the beat up and down his back (moderately gently!). Don't pound or tap on bony areas; stick to the areas that are well muscled. You can also slap with your palm, tap with your fingertips, or cup with your palm curled. Most people enjoy tapotement only for short periods of time, such as 30 seconds to a minute at most.

Back Off

The percussive strokes of tapotement are meant to be stimulating to the nervous system and increase circulation. They are not meant to be hard or painful, so it's best to start lightly and build up force gradually, checking in with the receiver as you do so. Use caution in the kidney area—below the last ribs and above the iliac crest. They are especially vulnerable to injury from a pounding that is too "enthusiastic."

4. After tapotement, always finish by smoothing his back and "making nice" with three or four effleurage strokes.

The Least You Need to Know

◆ A quick massage of the neck, shoulders, and back can be wonderful when you don't have time for a full massage.

◆ This quick massage can be done with the receiver seated almost anywhere.

◆ This massage requires a minimum of setup, and the only props needed are a chair and some pillows.

In This Chapter

- ◆ Relieving everyday neck tension

- ◆ Sensitivity is key in finding areas of tension

- ◆ Understanding the various positions possible for neck and shoulder massage

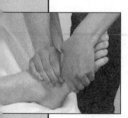
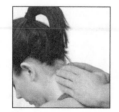
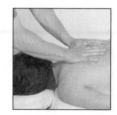
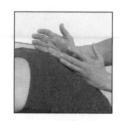
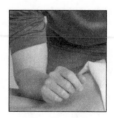
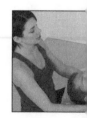

Chapter 7

The Neck, Shoulders, and Upper Back

Many of the strains of daily life produce tension and discomfort in the neck, shoulder, and upper back areas. By learning techniques to address specific upper body areas, you can reduce pain, stiffness, and stress-related tension. Developing sensitivity in palpating the neck and shoulder muscles helps you identify areas of tension in this area of the body and allows you to relieve that tension.

Neck, shoulder and upper back massage can be applied in a number of positions—supine, side-lying, and even standing.

Beginning on the Neck

We have to hold our heads up all day, and sometimes that can be a pain in the neck—literally! Getting a massage helps, but lying in the supine (face up) position while getting that massage is another story. The supine position is excellent for relaxation, stress relief, and the release of muscular tension.

Back Off

A stiff neck accompanied by a severe headache can signal serious illness. Do not massage a person with these symptoms. Send him to his doctor.

1. With your partner lying supine on a table, sit at his head. Start with a contact hold on his upper shoulders, your palms facing downward.

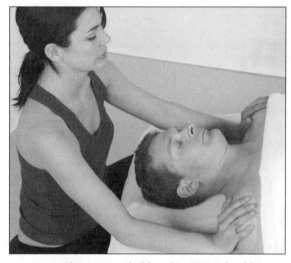

Begin with a contact hold on his upper shoulders.

2. Recognize and coordinate with his breathing pattern. You'll notice that within just five breaths, his breathing begins to slow simply under the calm weight of your hands.

3. With your palms against his skin, start just below his ears and perform effleurage strokes down both sides of his neck, out and around his deltoid muscles, rotating your hand outward so your palm remains on the back of his shoulders. Come toward the spine and pull your hands up the back of his neck.

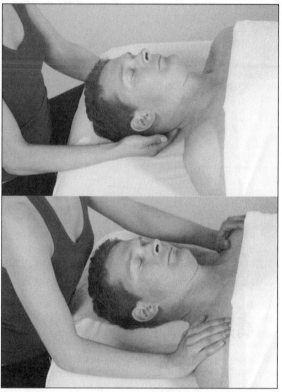

Begin your strokes on his neck just below his ears, and go all the way out around his shoulders and back up his neck.

4. Repeat a few times, exploring for areas of tension or holding as you make the strokes. If he tries to pick up his head as you make the stroke up the back of his neck, ask him to allow his head to be heavy in your hands and to concentrate on breathing into his belly.

5. Continue pulling strokes. As your hands come back around toward his spine, cup his neck with one entire hand and fingers. Lean back as you perform this to create the necessary stability required to keep his head from moving around as you do the pulling stroke.

Back Off

Avoid all work on the neck within 72 hours of any accident. The muscles might be tight and uncomfortable, and the receiver might want to gain some relief, but the muscles are doing an important job of splinting the injury while the neck is in its early stages of recovery. If there's any question about the severity of an injury, it's best to get a doctor's or chiropractor's assessment before you massage the area. It's also best to avoid working on a receiver's neck or back if he is under a physician's care for either acute or chronic orthopedic conditions. He should seek his doctor's permission to receive massage in these cases.

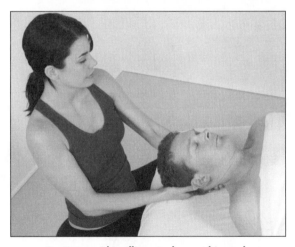

Continue with pulling strokes on his neck.

6. As your hand moves up his neck and the back of his head, your other hand should begin the same movement, taking the weight of his head and neck as your first hand returns to the bottom of his neck. This stroke, when performed smoothly and with a minimum of head and neck "bobbling," will feel like a continuous, flowing, smoothing, and stretching of chronically compressed and tight neck muscles.

7. At the end of the last repetition, allow your last hand stroke to "catch up" with the one on the back of his head, and hold his head in your hands as they rest on the working surface. Apply at least five or six of these strokes.

Press Here

Note that during the pulling stroke, your hands should be sliding on the working surface and the receiver's head should not be lifted any higher than necessary to allow your hands to glide up his neck. This is a nice stroke to insert between other strokes whenever you're massaging the head, face, and neck. Consider it a "chorus" of lengthening effleurage, or apply five or six of these strokes between other parts of the sequence.

8. With your hands, fingers up, on your partner's upper shoulder muscles, lean forward and use your body weight to sink into the muscles. Direct the pressure toward his feet. Sink in on his exhalation, and ease off the pressure on his inhalations. Your hands will move from near his neck out to the point of his shoulders. Apply one or two of these strokes, going out to the shoulders and then coming back close in to the neck. Your hands should both press at the same time, as alternating pressure from hand to hand puts some strain on the alignment of the cervical *vertebrae*.

Definition

The **vertebrae** (singular *vertebra*) are the small individual bones that make up the spinal column, which runs from the base of the skull down to the sacrum. The spinal column is divided into three parts: the cervical vertebrae, which make up the neck, the thoracic vertebrae, which make up the thorax or chest, and the lumbar vertebrae, which make up the lower back.

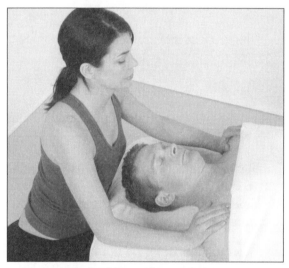

Move to his shoulders and use palming pressure.

Do not perform this move if you have any discomfort with your wrists in the hyperextended position, and do not apply excess force when doing the palming in any case, to protect your wrists; it is a gentle move.

Circular Friction Along the Base of the Skull

The muscles on each side of the spine in the neck, the posterior cervical region, are under constant strain from carrying the weight of the head. Many of the activities of daily life add additional stress to the neck; maintaining a certain angle of the neck to see a computer screen

or driving a car in bad weather conditions are two common culprits in stressing the muscles in the back of the neck. Circular friction allows you to palpate for areas of tension and loosen those areas at the same time.

1. With your palms facing up, make small, mirror-image finger circles just to each side of his spine. Allow your hands to move up and down his neck, always staying clear of the spinous processes of the vertebrae and exploring for areas of tension. Do this for 20 seconds or more.

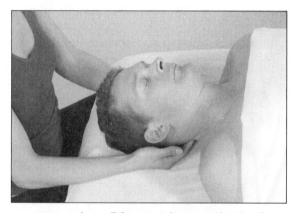

Begin with small finger circles on each side of his neck.

At Your Fingertips

Depending on the amount of muscle tension you feel, you might want to perform circular friction combined with the next strokes for 2 or 3 minutes to really help these tense muscles relax.

2. Continue the circles back and forth across the base of his skull (occipital ridge) until you feel tension in the area begin to melt.

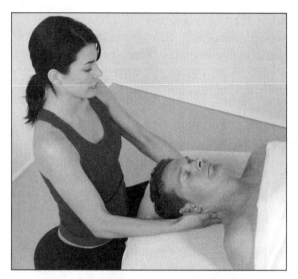

Apply circular friction with your fingers along the base of the skull.

About 20 muscles are located in this small area at the base of the skull, and as you increase your sensitivity, you'll begin to find many nuances of texture and tone in them. It might be helpful to close your eyes to intensify the focus on the feeling and sensitivity in your hands. Remember to allow your fingers to just rest for several seconds on areas that might be willing to release tension and melt. The receiver might sigh after you've had your still hands on him in this way for a few of his breaths. This can effect a profound release of tension.

The Side of the Neck

Stretching the neck to one side while applying lengthening strokes can help bring a feeling of length back into a person's neck that feels tight and compressed. Anyone who talks on the phone with the receiver between his shoulder and his ear will especially benefit from the lengthening these strokes provide.

1. Taking the back of the receiver's head in your left hand, gently tilt his head to the left side, bringing his ear closer to his shoulder.

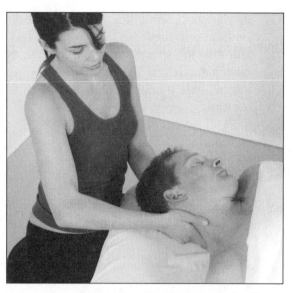

After turning his head to the side, begin with effleurage on the side of his neck.

2. Allow his head to continue to rest in your left palm, which will keep it in place as your right hand begins an effleurage stroke below his ear and comes all the way down his neck and shoulder, around his deltoid, and back up to the starting point on the side of his neck. Repeat this three or four times, focusing on the nice stretch that's produced as you slowly lengthen the side of his neck and shoulder.

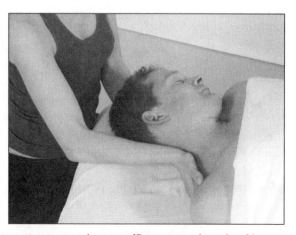

Continue with more effleurage on the side of his neck, moving down to his shoulders and back up again.

3. Repeat on the other side. Be sure to move his head very slowly and smoothly as you take it from a stretch on one side to the other side. Return his head to the center, and hold it in both hands for a few breaths.

Back Off _____

Never pull the neck into an extreme side stretch. When taking the receiver's head over to one side, move very slowly so you can sense when you're reaching his neck's range-of-motion limit. Stop slightly before you get to his end point for the stretch.

Effleurage on the Side of the Neck

Start with effleurage down the sides of his neck, around his shoulders, and up the back of his neck three or four times, just as you did to start the sequence.

You might want to throw in a few pulling strokes on his neck as well before closing the area with a contact hold, with your hands either on his shoulders or holding his head in your palms.

Side-Lying Massage on the Neck and Shoulders

For receivers who are 22 weeks or more pregnant or who have lower back problems that make supine and prone positions uncomfortable, working in the side-lying position can be a good option. Some people get stuffy noses when they lie face down and are more comfortable side-lying. In addition, the side-lying position allows greater access to both hips and shoulders, and more options are possible to create movement in the joints. Many people sleep in this position because it is so comfortable, and will simply enjoy it more than other positions, relaxing more completely during the massage.

The side-lying position is an especially good position for exploring (palpating) the area around the shoulder blade (scapula). You can increase access to the areas where muscles attach to the bone by using one hand on the deltoid to move the scapula toward where the other hand is exploring along the edge of the bone with circular friction.

At Your Fingertips _____

All work in this section is done on one side and then repeated on the other side after the receiver turns over.

1. Place a pillow large enough to keep the receiver's neck in alignment with the back under his head and neck. Place another between his ankles and knees, and offer a third "huggy pillow" to keep his upper arm in a supported neutral position, so it isn't hanging down in front of his chest or belly.

2. While seated behind the receiver, apply petrissage to one side of his upper shoulder (trapezius) and deltoid area. Alternate the lifting and squeezing actions between both hands, feeding the muscles from one palm to the other. Perform this action for about 30 or 40 seconds before moving on to the next step.

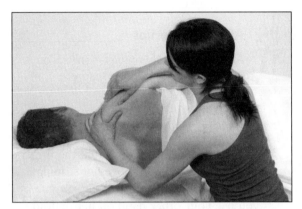

Begin with petrissage on the upper shoulder and deltoid areas.

3. Locate the entire border of the scapula, softening the muscle attachments with circular friction as you go. This might require anywhere from 1 to 3 minutes, depending on how thoroughly you're exploring the area around the scapula and how many areas of muscle tightness you find.

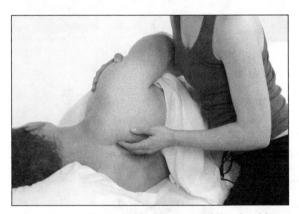

Continue with circular friction around his shoulder blade.

4. Using an oscillating vibration that comes from your shoulder and down your arm through your palm, move all around the whole shoulder area, watching how the vibration ripples out into the muscles. This is a demanding stroke for the person performing the massage, and it is unlikely that you will want to perform it for more than about 20 seconds.

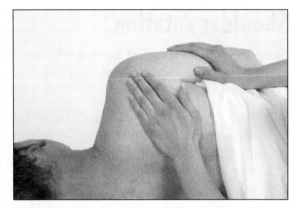

Apply oscillating vibration to the upper shoulder.

Press Here

This vibrating action is confusing to the muscles and often induces greater relaxation, even more than more targeted and deeper friction. If an area shows less rippling moving through it, explore it with your fingers and see if some more circular friction helps it release tension.

While you're producing vibration in the muscles with one hand, lay the other hand, which we call the "mother hand," on the hip or back—anywhere that's comfortable for both of you. Receivers unconsciously like to know what the hand you're not actively using is doing, and its passive weight on his body is comforting.

Back Off

If there's redness and a feverish feeling in any area of the body, such as in the area of the shoulder joint, this is an indication that the receiver may have localized inflammation. Areas of inflammation show that the body has mobilized its forces to attack an infection or to promote healing of an injury. Leave areas of inflammation strictly alone, saving massage for further along in the recovery process.

Shoulder Rotation

Shoulder rotations are great for loosening up and increasing mobility in the receiver's shoulders and upper arms.

1. Facing the receiver's head, reach under her arm and cup your hand around her deltoid muscle, with her upper arm supported on your arm.

2. Place your other hand just above her scapula, and rotate her shoulder up toward her ear, back toward you, down, and then forward. Experiment with the motion, going slowly so you can feel for restrictions in range of motion without pushing the limits too far.

☝ **At Your Fingertips**

Anytime you perform joint mobilization movements, go very slowly so you can sense when you're moving a limb to the edge of its range of motion.

3. After about five rotations, hold the fingers of the hand that was above her scapula along the middle border of her scapula as you use your other hand on her deltoid to press her shoulder back onto your fingers.

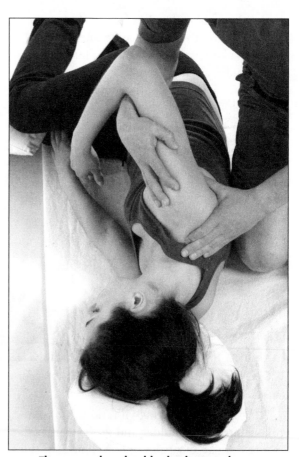

Then rotate her shoulder back toward you.

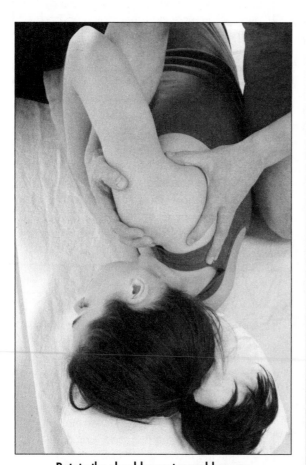

Rotate the shoulder up toward her ear.

Back Off

If the receiver has limited range of motion in her shoulder, especially if it is accompanied by pain and difficulty in making normal movements, she might have a torn rotator cuff muscle. Advise her to seek medical advice rather than massage.

4. Gradually move your fingers up and down the edge of her scapula, creating pressure with your other hand throughout the process.

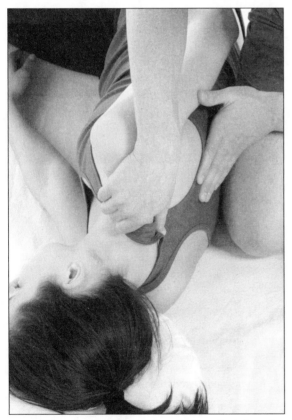

Move your fingers up and down along the edge of her scapula.

Deep Effleurage of the Deltoid Muscle

The deltoid muscle plays a key role in movements of the arm at the shoulder, and because this muscle has portions on the front, sides, and back of the shoulders, it performs a lot of different actions. Reaching, throwing, lifting, and all racquet sports put a load on these hardworking shoulder muscles. Massage can assist in the process of relieving post-game soreness and returning the arm to pain-free optimal function quickly.

1. Still holding her shoulder as for shoulder rotation, with the hand that was on the border of her scapula, start gliding it deeply up the back of her upper arm and all the way to the point of her shoulder.

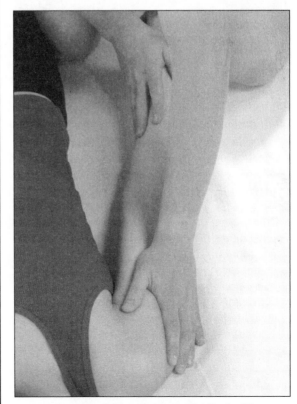

Progress to gliding strokes on the back of her upper arm.

2. Continue to make these strokes in the same direction, gradually working around toward the front of her arm and shoulder. It should take about six strokes to get all the way around the front of the shoulder.

3. When you reach a point where it becomes awkward, support her shoulder with your hand that's been gliding, and continue your strokes with the hand that's been holding her deltoid.

4. Finish by making four to six deep gliding strokes from the point of her shoulder up the side of her neck as you hold the shoulder to put a nice stretch on the side of her neck.

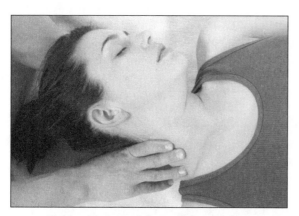

Finish with several deep, gliding strokes.

Back Off

Most people are aware if they have shoulders that are easily dislocated. Understand that they may not be comfortable with motions that move the arm around if they have suffered dislocations in the past. It is best to simply avoid shoulder joint mobilization moves for those who have had dislocations.

Standing

When you just have a few minutes to spare and the receiver could use some loosening up of the shoulders and back, a brief dressed standing sequence can be just the ticket.

1. Standing behind the receiver, begin by applying tapotement on his upper shoulders, moving back and forth from the base of his neck to his outer shoulders, with one hand on each side of the spine. Avoid making percussive strokes directly on bony areas.

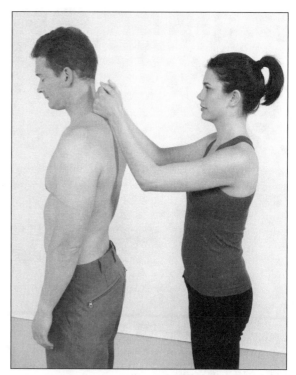

Begin standing massage with tapotement on his upper shoulders.

2. Direct the receiver to bow his head forward, gradually rolling downward, starting at his neck, then his mid-back, and finally all the way to his lower back.

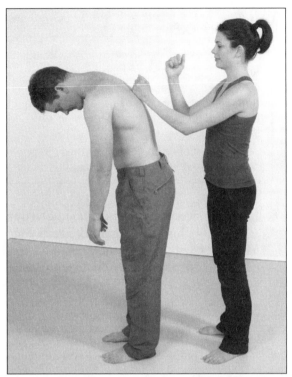

Continue with tapotement on his back while he bends forward.

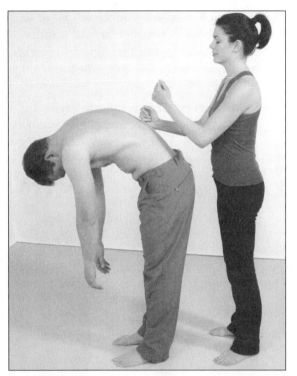

The receiver controls how long you apply tapotement to any area by rolling forward as you work.

3. As he moves, continue your tapotement on his back, keeping your hands in roughly the same position but striking different areas of the back as he rolls forward. By bending, he can control how long you apply tapotement to a particular area of his back.

Back Off

This might not be a good massage sequence to practice if the receiver has dizziness or balance problems. He could hurt himself if he pitches forward or falls over while rolling forward.

4. When he has rolled all the way forward and you can reach his lower back, switch to tapotement back and forth across his hip (ilium) area. Keep a consistent tempo with your strokes.

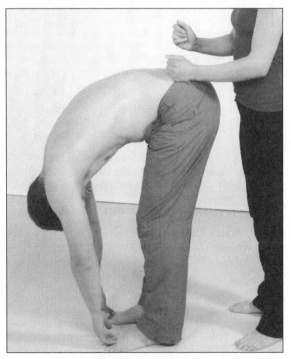

With the receiver bent all the way forward, you can continue with tapotement on his hips.

5. Continue the percussive strokes for as long as he wishes to remain in a bent position. As he gradually rolls back up and straightens, your strokes will cover the areas of his middle and upper back.

6. When he's completely upright again, repeat the tapotement across his shoulders for about 20 to 30 seconds.

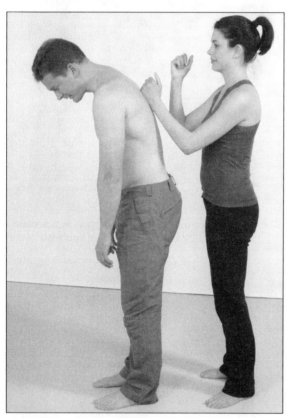

As the receiver gradually rolls back up, you can reach his shoulders again for more tapotement.

7. Apply at least a dozen lifting and squeezing strokes on both sides of his upper shoulders, either bringing the thumbs and heels of your hands forward toward your fingers on the fronts of the shoulders or bringing your fingers back toward your thumbs. (Each of these strokes has a different feel, so you may want to ask your receiver which he prefers.)

Back Off

Do not cross the spine as you're doing tapotement; steer clear of the spinous processes of the vertebrae. Thin people who do not have heavy muscles over the scapula will appreciate a light tapotement over their scapulae as well. Also, avoid heavy percussive strokes on the kidney area, just below the ribs, and above the hips.

8. Finish by sweeping down the body. Starting at the top of his receiver's head, sweep your hands very lightly down the sides of his face, neck, shoulders, and back. Squat down as you bring the feathery, light, sweeping stroke all the way to his feet. Repeat three times.

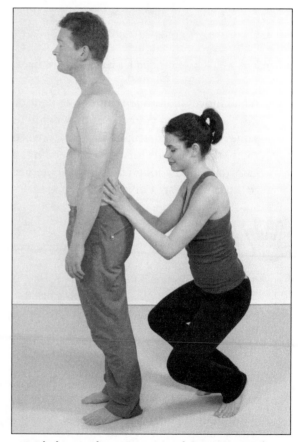

Finish the standing massage with sweeping strokes from the top of his head all the way to his feet.

The Least You Need to Know

◆ The neck, shoulders, and upper back are some of the main places people hold their tensions from daily life. A massage to this area can do the receiver a world of good.

◆ This area of the body can be massaged with the receiver supine (face up), side-lying, or even standing.

◆ Shoulder rotation can increase flexibility in the shoulders, neck, and upper arms.

In This Chapter

◆ Simple techniques to relax arms and hands

◆ Positions for arm and hand massage

◆ The best strokes for hands, fingers, and arms

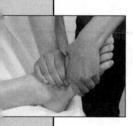
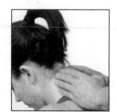
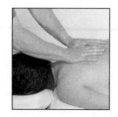
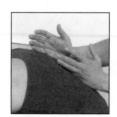
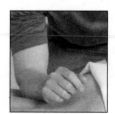
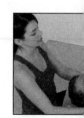

Chapter 8

The Arms and Hands

We use our arms and hands constantly at work and at play, and often we only notice how much we use them when we have a painful injury or condition that keeps us from using an arm or hand. Because these areas of the body get so much use (and abuse), getting a hand or arm massage can be a wonderful, relaxing way to spend a few minutes.

The Best Positions for Hand and Arm Massage

The hand and arm massage in this chapter assumes that the receiver is relaxed in the supine position, but you can also do hand and arm massage on a seated person. It's not quite as relaxing as when he's supine, but it's still great for tired arms and hands.

To do a seated hand and arm massage, you and the receiver should sit close together in chairs. Place a pillow in the receiver's lap for him to rest his elbow on. It takes a little improvisation to apply the strokes, but one of the beauties of elbows, shoulders, and wrists is that they move in many directions, making it easy to adjust the receiver's hands and arms and keep your hands and arms in a relatively neutral position while you perform the massage. If you're giving a seated massage, you can rest the receiver's elbow on the pillow, his hand on your thigh, etc., to achieve the same effect.

Arm and hand massage can also be performed effectively on a person in the side-lying position. If he's lying on his right side, place his left arm along his left side and hip, and work his arm, hand, and shoulder from a standing position. Then, he can turn over and you can repeat on his other side. Be sure to massage his entire arm and hand before moving on to the other side.

Back Off

You don't work on hands and arms in the prone (face-down) position because you aren't able to move the forearm and hand for easy access. The elbow simply doesn't bend that way. Also, it's best to minimize the amount of time you have a person in the prone position because it can lead to a stuffy nose.

Working on the Hand

We often take our hands for granted, but they are truly wonders of nature in their fine dexterity, allowing us to do incredibly delicate activities such as threading a tiny needle with fine thread, as well as activities requiring great grip strength and agility. Most of us spend a majority of our work and hobby time performing tasks with our hands that require endless repetitions of the same basic moves, and over time, this can cause discomfort or injury. Massage of the hands not only relaxes them and decreases pain, but it can also improve the receiver's awareness of his hands so he can learn to use them in ways that help maintain hand health and dexterity.

1. Begin with a contact hold, standing or seated beside the receiver, with one of your hands on his shoulder and the other on his hand. Get in touch with his breath, breathing with him for three to five breaths.

2. Perform long, gliding effleurage strokes from your partner's fingertips all the way around his shoulder, using your hand closest to his hip to secure his hand on the surface he's lying on so you're not pushing his shoulder up toward his ear with the stroke. About four or five long effleurage strokes allow you to evenly spread the cream or lotion over his entire arm, begin to warm up the muscles, and explore where he might be holding tension in his arm and hand.

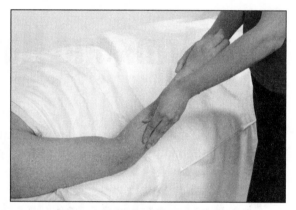

Begin with long gliding strokes from his fingertips up his arm.

Press Here

People often have hangnails, cuts, and other injuries on their hands. Look for such injuries and be alert about working close to injured areas. The hands and fingers contain a large number of nerves, making them especially sensitive to pain. Similarly, arthritis is common in hands, and you must be alert to swollen, hot, and painful joints in the fingers when you're massaging this area.

3. Place your thumbs on the back of his hand with your fingers curled under his palm, his hand at a level comfortable for you, and his elbow resting on the table.

Squeeze first on one side and then on the other as you slide your hands toward the end of his thumb and little finger.

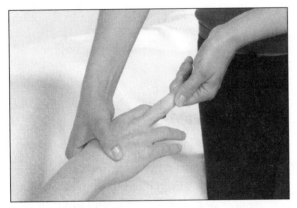

Move on to pulling stroke with twist on middle finger.

4. Accentuate your side-to-side movement at his wrist as you do the milking stroke on his hand. This enhances the smoothness of rotation of his wrist. The focus of this stroke is on the areas to each side of his palm, the same part of your hand that's most important in this stroke. Continue for about 20 seconds and then repeat on his other hand.

 Back Off

Don't try to turn his palm face up while his elbow is straight at his side. This puts the elbow in an uncomfortable bind. The elbow is designed to rotate out away from the body in this position.

5. Holding his hand in yours, squeeze his fingers one by one between the thumb and fingers of your other hand. Add a little twist as you go from the base to the tip of his fingers, once or twice per finger.

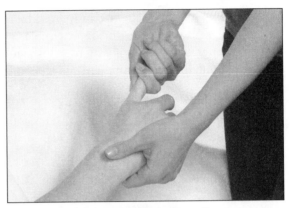

Work on the fingers individually, with a squeeze, slide, and twist.

At Your Fingertips

Some people think the squeeze, slide, and twist move should pop the joints of the fingers, but don't exert that much pressure. If you're working moderately and a joint or two does pop, it's nothing to worry about. It's just not the goal of this move.

6. With your thumbs on the back of his hand pointing toward his wrist, spread out the top of his hand toward his palm, squeezing his palm in on itself. Reverse the motion to stretch his palm and open it up. Do this about three times in each direction.

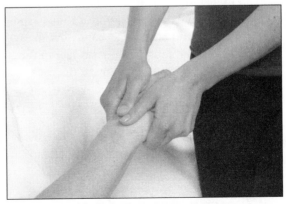

Move from his fingers to spreading strokes on the top of his hand.

7. Holding his arm, palm up, away from his body, spread the palm and apply circular friction with your thumbs all over his palm for about 20 to 30 seconds.

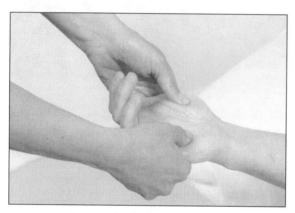

Finish with circular friction on his palm.

You can apply friction vigorously on the palms because our hands are used to such force in our day-to-day activities. Our palms are used much of the time for grasping and holding things, so stretching the palm in the opposite direction is delightful.

Massaging the Forearm

Many of the muscles that perform the actions of our hands are located in our forearms, so the same stresses that can affect our hands can cause pain and tension in our forearms. Because of the size of the forearm, it's an easy area to massage, even for those who have small hands. Notice how many distinct muscles you can feel in the forearm as you massage it; many of the muscles have areas of tightness and soreness that you can palpate and release.

1. With his elbow still resting on the table, hold his hand with one of your hands. With your other hand, begin squeezing effleurage toward his elbow about six or eight times, alternating the area of his arm you're squeezing by switching your hands from time to time.

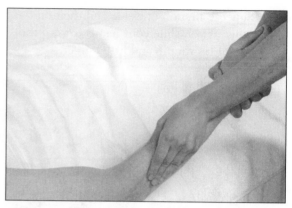

Start with squeezing effleurage from wrist to elbow.

2. Keep your hand on his arm as you glide it back toward his hand, but remember that the force of the stroke should be from his wrist toward his elbow, toward his heart. As you perform the stroke, be conscious of any tight areas and linger there with more strokes, or simply stop your stroke and apply compression for several seconds.

At Your Fingertips

Be sure to have your hand leading with your thumb and forefinger rather than the pinkie side of your hand. This protects you from putting the wrong kind of pressure on your wrist and possibly injuring it.

3. With his arm in the same position, apply lifting and squeezing petrissage on areas of his forearm where you found tightness and tension for 20 to 30 seconds.

You can also do some rotating "Indian rub" friction around his arm. This can feel really nice with adequate lubrication, especially around the wrist area.

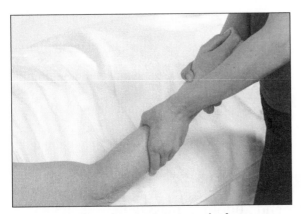

Move to kneading petrissage on the forearm.

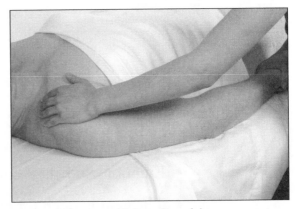

Finish the arm with kneading of the upper arm and shoulders.

Kneading the Upper Arm

The muscles of the upper arm are larger and stronger than those of the forearm. The biceps, a muscle most of us are acquainted with from arm-wrestling is a good example. We use these muscles for larger movements than those we make with the forearms, and for actions that require greater strength. They can become sore and overtaxed from repeated lifting. Often these muscles feel very tired in addition to feeling achy. Massage can flush away the by-products of muscle contraction and renew the muscles with fresh nutrients and oxygen.

1. After placing his arm and hand back on the surface, move around to sit at his head. This enables you to easily reach both of his shoulders at the same time.

2. Reach forward and knead his upper arms and shoulders on both sides for a minute or two.

3. You might want to smooth his shoulder area by doing three or four effleurage and pulling strokes on his neck here to complete the sequence.

4. Finish with contact hold on his shoulders.

Back Off

Use only a very light pressure on the arm of someone who has had lymph nodes in the breast or armpit area removed. Even the pressure of a blood pressure cuff should be avoided for these people.

The Least You Need to Know

◆ Our hands and arms are used more in our daily lives than most other parts of our bodies.

◆ Simple techniques can relax arms and hands and relieve the tension that comes from daily use.

◆ Arm and hand massage can be done with the receiver lying supine, side-lying, or sitting in a chair.

◆ Repetitive actions with the hands and arms can lead to discomforts that massage can reduce.

In This Chapter

- ◆ Emotions and chest and abdomen massage
- ◆ The gentle touch for chest and abdomen massage
- ◆ Men and women are different
- ◆ Special techniques for the abdomen

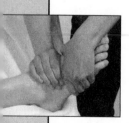
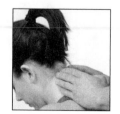
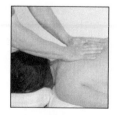
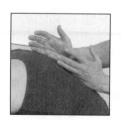
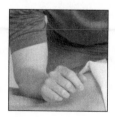
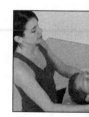

Chapter 9

The Chest and Abdomen

Massage of the chest can be good for helping to loosen tight muscles that round the shoulders forward. Rounded shoulders can create pain in the upper back if the pectoral muscles of the chest are so strong that they stretch out the back muscles, massage of the chest can aid in relieving upper back pain as well as any discomfort in the chest area itself.

Abdominal massage, though frequently overlooked in massage sessions, can be useful for tension held in the belly, either from stress or from the habit of holding in your belly to look trim in your midsection.

Understanding His Emotional Release

We tend to think of our emotions as being something in our minds, and certainly we can feed emotional reactions by dwelling on certain thoughts or memories. But if you think about it, you might recognize that many of the physical sensations associated with emotions are experienced in the chest and abdomen. Have "gut reactions"? Ever experienced a "broken heart"?

The chemicals associated with emotions have many more receptor sites in the abdomen and chest than we have in our brains. (Think of receptor sites as the locks and the chemicals —neurotransmitters—as keys to fit those locks.) Because of this, we tend to store emotions in this area, and because many of us are seldom touched there, it's not uncommon to have those emotions stored in this area rise to the surface when caring massage is performed on the chest and abdomen. Frequently these emotions come to the surface in the form of tears, but occasionally other emotions, like laughter, may arise as well.

Press Here _____

It's important for your partner to feel that he can safely experience and express whatever he's feeling during the massage. He needs to be able to trust you and know that you're holding a nonjudgmental space for any expression of his emotional response to the massage.

You can respond to this kind of situation in a few ways. You can let his emotions flow through without comment or ask him if he'd like for you to stop the massage if the emotions seem too intense. You might simply offer a tissue or rest a calm hand on his shoulder until the emotional release passes. Emotional release can be very cleansing for your partner.

Working on the Upper Chest

This massage is done with your partner lying supine on a massage table or on the floor. Begin by standing or sitting at his shoulder.

Back Off _____

If a person has swelling, nausea, vomiting or chest pains, massage is not appropriate for him at the time. He should seek medical care instead.

1. First perform a slow effleurage stroke across his upper chest just beneath his clavicles. Reduce pressure at the recipient's mid-chest over the sternum.

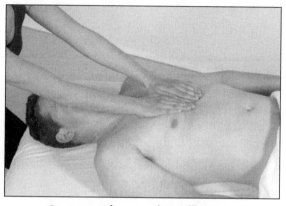

Start out with upper chest effleurage.

2. Moving to his head, place your hands just below his clavicles, and do three or four spreading effleurage strokes toward his armpits, bringing the stroke over and around his deltoids, across the back of his shoulders, and up the back of his neck.

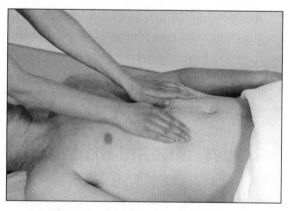

Bilateral spreading strokes come next.

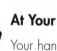

At Your Fingertips _____

Your hands do a lot of rotating here, so don't exert too much pressure, or you could harm your wrists. Also, it can be quite uncomfortable for men to have their chest hair pulled during a massage. Be sure to use extra lotion, cream, or oil when you are massaging especially hairy areas.

3. Move your strokes on the chest out toward his armpits. The front margin of the armpit, where the *pectoral muscle* goes under the deltoid, is used a lot and can definitely benefit from massage. (But beware of working the hollow of the armpit. It's full of blood vessels, lymph nodes, and nerves that are close to the surface. Besides, many people have ticklish armpits.)

Definition

The **pectoral muscles** are the large muscles that run from the breastbone (sternum) out to the humerus and under the front edges of the deltoid muscles. Sometimes we hear athletes referring to these two large muscles as their "pecs." They are used in many shoulder and arm movements.

---

4. On a man, continue with effleurage down the center of his chest and abdomen, rotating your hands outward at his waist. Follow this by performing a pulling stroke back up his sides, ending at the center of his chest. Then continue the stroke all the way around his shoulders and up his neck as in the previous movement. Repeat two or three more times.

When massaging the chest, avoid breast tissue (including nipples on men) unless you are a licensed or certified professional with advanced training in breast massage. Most chest and abdomen massage is done in the supine position, although it may be adapted for the side-lying position as well. You might not be able to do upper chest effleurage on some women because their breast tissue rises up to their clavicles when they are supine.

Moving On to the Abdomen

Your partner might not feel comfortable receiving abdominal massage because he's unhappy with the shape and size of his belly, or he might be afraid of being tickled. No one should ever feel coerced into receiving massage on the abdominal area. If he can give it a try, though, your partner will be likely to find he enjoys this part of a massage session.

Similarly, you might feel hesitant to offer abdominal massage, but when you become accustomed to it, you'll find that both you and your partner can enjoy massage in the area that's considered the "seat of the emotions."

1. On a man (or a woman covered by a drape across her breast area), perform six to eight large clockwise circles of effleurage on the abdomen.

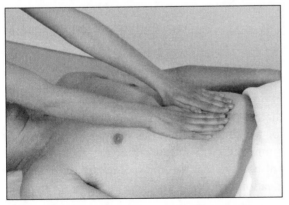

On a man, you can continue with effleurage down the center of his chest and to the abdomen.

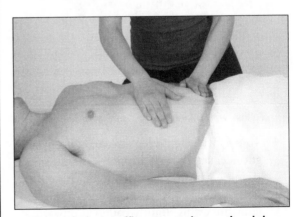

Use large, clockwise effleurage strokes on the abdomen.

Press Here _____

It's important to work in a clockwise direction on the abdomen, because that's the direction food moves in the intestines.

2. Follow with raking strokes on abdomen, either on one side of the chest and abdomen or both at once. Raking strokes open the lower back area as well as work the abdomen and ribcage areas. For one-sided raking, stand or sit at the recipient's side near his waist, and reach across his body, putting your hands well under his opposite side. Your hands should be in back of his waist, pulling toward you (and his midline) first with one hand and then the other.

3. Create an endless flowing and lifting feeling with this alternating hand-pulling. Move your strokes up the side of his body toward his armpit and then back down, all the way into his hip area. This will probably require eight strokes or so to move up his side and back down to his hip.

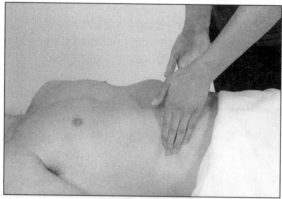

Follow with raking strokes on the abdomen.

4. To perform the raking stroke on both sides at once, stand or sit at the recipient's side, facing his head, and reach under his each side of his back with your hands, bringing your fingertips slightly rounded upward,

near his spine. Pull and rake your hands across his lower back and then around his sides toward the center front of his belly two or three times. Two or three repetitions are about all you'll probably want to do. Expect your partner to want more than that!

5. End with a contact hold with one hand on his abdomen just below his naval and your other hand over his heart for four or five breaths.

At Your Fingertips _____

This can be a challenging stroke for you to perform, depending on your size relative to your partner's size, and your height relative to the surface the receiver is resting on. You might want to brace your thighs against the table, if you're working on one, or kneel if you're working on the floor.

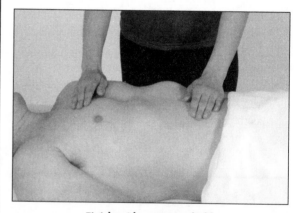

Finish with a contact hold.

All abdomen massage should be fairly light in pressure. There are many medical conditions that might not be apparent in the early stages for which deep abdominal massage is not recommended. If you're working and feel a strong pulse, leave that specific spot and try another location nearby.

Back Off

Watch out for hardware when massaging the abdomen. Pulling a belly button ring could quickly ruin your partner's relaxation.

The Least You Need to Know

◆ Chest and abdomen massage can provoke a powerful emotional reaction.

◆ Abdominal massage requires a lighter touch than massage on many other parts of the body.

◆ Men and women need to be treated differently during chest massage.

◆ Always work on the abdomen in a clockwise direction.

In This Chapter

- ◆ The leg defined
- ◆ Milking strokes on the foot
- ◆ Point compression on the foot
- ◆ Don't forget the knee

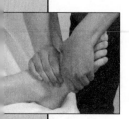
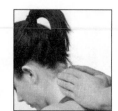
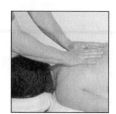
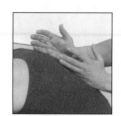
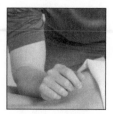
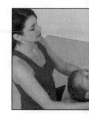

Chapter 10

Thighs, Legs, and Feet

Whether you're on your feet all day or just need a leg or foot massage, you've come to the right chapter. Before we get in to the hands-on techniques, though, let's look at some massage terminology so you know exactly what we're talking about. In technical massage terminology …

- The *thigh* is the area between the knee and the hip/groin area.
- The *leg* is the area between the knee and the ankle.

Keep this in mind, as that's the terminology we use throughout this chapter.

Effleurage from Foot to Hip

Most of this massage sequence is applied to the front of the leg and thigh, with your partner in a relaxed, face up (supine) position. You do all the movements on one foot, leg, and thigh and then repeat on the other side. When working on the backs of the legs, of course your partner must be in the prone position.

Due to space considerations, we've used photographs showing work on the back of legs in this chapter. Remember that you will be working on both sides of the leg, and the strokes on the front of the legs are generally similar to those used on the back of the legs. See the DVD for more information.

Back Off

You shouldn't be working on a pregnant woman if she isn't your partner, and even then, you need to get further information about massaging her. Deep venous thrombosis is much more common in pregnant women, as are varicosities, and other leg conditions warrant caution as well. Certain points in her lower legs and feet can stimulate contractions and should not be massaged before the baby is full term.

1. Begin with contact hold on your partner's leg. Hold for four or five of her breaths.

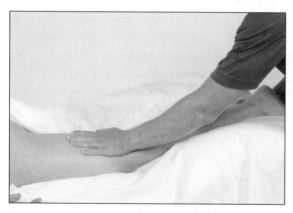

Start out with a contact hold.

2. Face her upper body, and use three to six effleurage strokes to spread the lubricant from her toes all the way around her hip. You might need to apply additional cream or lotion, especially in winter; many people have very dry skin on their feet and legs.

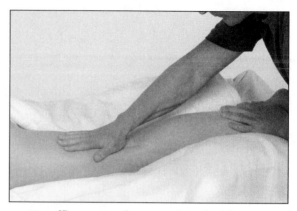

Use effleurage strokes to work in the lubricant.

Press Here

If you see blue and elevated veins in the legs, these are likely varicose veins. Never put moderate or deep pressure on a varicose vein. Spider veins, on the other hand, are reddish and are not raised. These present no problem for receiving massage.

3. As you apply effleurage to the foot, leg, and thigh, you are connecting them for your partner, and it gives you the opportunity to warm the muscle tissue and to explore the area for tightness. Consider lingering on any tight areas you find before moving on, perhaps suggesting to your partner that she focus her breath into the area and allow the tension to melt away.

4. Taking her foot closest to you in both your hands, perform a series of about 10 strong, short pulling effleurage strokes first on one side of her foot and then the other. Your strokes should be alternately lengthening each side of her foot.

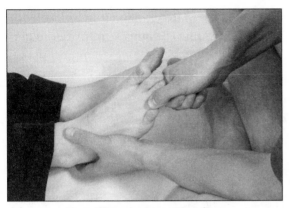

Use milking strokes on her foot.

5. Then reverse the action, pushing toward her heel on the arch and the outside of her foot, moving gradually into circles on the front of her ankle. Always remember to exert more pressure as you massage toward the heart than when you massage in the opposite direction. Small, one-way valves help the blood flow back to the heart and lungs rather than pooling in the extremities, and these valves may be damaged by downward (against-the-flow) pressure.

6. Place your thumbs on the bottom of her foot, with your fingers over the top of her foot. Perform circular friction all over the sole of her foot, paying special attention to her arch, for 30 seconds or so.

7. With your thumbs, press into points along her foot, feeling for tight or dense areas. Don't be surprised if some points you press cause her to report sensations somewhere else in her body. These are reflex effects and form the basis for reflexology, a specialized form of massage.

 Back Off _____

Many people, especially athletes, have bruises, swelling, cuts, strains, and sprains of the leg, ankle, knee, and thigh areas. Stay well away from sites of such injuries when performing a massage.

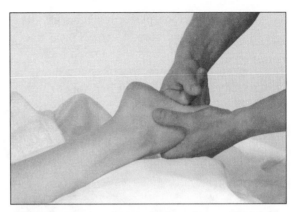

Use point compression on the foot along with circular friction.

8. "Indian rub" on feet and ankles Standing or sitting between her feet, take her foot into your hand so your thumbs and fingers are on the arch side of her foot. Then, wring her foot with both hands. This feels good when the skin is lubricated with lotion or cream.

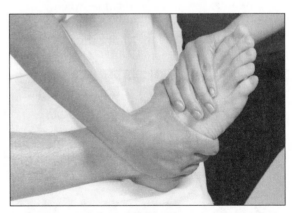

Wringing—along with lubrication—is great on the feet and ankles.

9. Move back and forth to different areas of her foot with the wringing action. You could even continue up her ankle and lower leg area with this stroke. Do not exceed 1 minute for this series of strokes, as it can be hard on your wrists.

10. To keep the rest of your partner's leg and thigh from feeling left out after all this

work on her foot, perform a "chorus" of three or four effleurage strokes on her entire leg, thigh, and foot again. This repeats the effleurage strokes you did at the beginning, ending at her upper thigh.

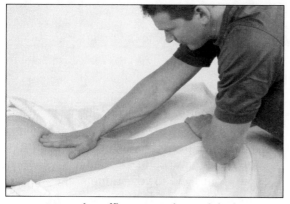

Proceed to effleurage on leg and thigh.

11. Facing your partner's side, begin to lift and squeeze her thigh muscles, feeding the muscles back and forth between your hands for about a minute, moving your hands to massage the entire thigh.

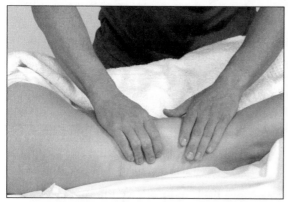

Next, apply petrissage strokes to her thigh.

12. Smooth out her thigh with effleurage, starting from knee to thigh for three to five strokes and then continuing with less pressure (away from her heart). Finish by gliding down to her foot, and with increased pressure, use effleurage—one hand chasing the other—in strokes up her thigh again.

Back Off _____

Be sure to keep the full surface of your palms on her muscles as you squeeze her thigh muscles. Otherwise, it might feel "pinchy" to her. Pinchy does not equal relaxation.

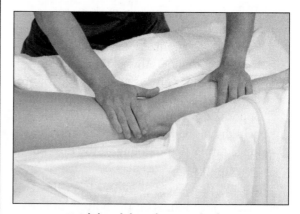

Finish by gliding down to the foot.

13. In the same position, place your hands with thumbs together on her thigh. Move your hands apart and down the inside and outside surfaces of her thigh, spreading her muscles. Continue this action, moving down her thigh and then down her leg to her foot, performing the spreading stroke as you go. (It's fine to apply the spreading stroke starting at her thigh and moving away from her torso, because the force of the stroke is outward rather than downward and won't damage the valves in her leg veins.) It will take at least 10 or 12 spreading strokes to traverse the length of her thigh and leg.

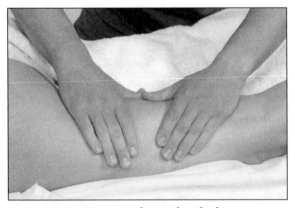

Petrissage strokes on her thigh.

14. Make an effleurage stroke back up to her knee, and place your hands on each side of her knee, with the little finger (*ulnar*) side of your hand against the sides of her knee. Move your hands in circles around her knee about a dozen repetitions—as if opening a jar with both hands. You could also apply small circular friction strokes with your fingers all around her kneecap.

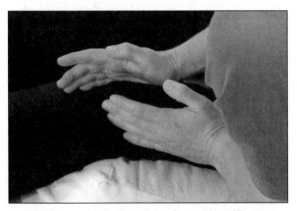

Don't leave out the knee! Apply circular effleurage around the kneecap.

15. Finally, connect the entire limb together with three or four more effleurage strokes from foot through thigh.

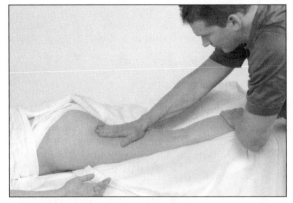

Finish by connecting the entire limb with effleurage strokes.

Back Off

If your partner has heat, redness, and pain in her leg, especially if she has been inactive, it may be a sign of deep venous thrombosis, and massaging her leg might cause a blood clot to break loose and move to her heart on lungs. A good rule of thumb for this and all other questionable conditions is "when in doubt, don't massage."

The Least You Need to Know

- In massage terminology, your leg is from your knee to your foot.
- The foot is uniquely connected to the rest of the body, and massage of the foot can produce sensations elsewhere in the body.
- Many muscle attachments and nerves are located in the knee area. Massage here can be beneficial in numerous ways.
- Massaging the foot, leg, and thigh connects the whole limb for your partner.

In This Chapter

- ◆ Ahhh ... back rubs
- ◆ Pinning and stretching
- ◆ Alternate back rub positions

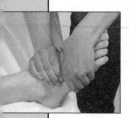
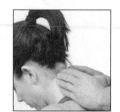
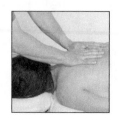
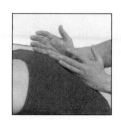
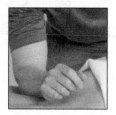
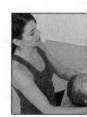

Chapter 11

The Back

Some of the largest contributors to lost time from work are back pain and injury. We know of several people who suffer from back pain, and you probably do, too. A back massage can help relieve some of that back tension. In fact, it's probably the most commonly thought-of type of massage.

Before you get started, know that some back pain and tension should not be massaged. Any back injury, particularly those that affect the spine, should not be massaged. Refer your partner to a physician if you're unsure.

But most regular back aches and pains come from muscles that have been overused, strained, or are reacting to poor postural habits. Massage of an aching back often can result in a lot of relief.

First Touch

Generally, you will have massaged much of your partner in the supine position before you get to his back. By the time he turns over into the prone position to receive massage on his back he will be relaxed and may even fall asleep, so consider using long, slow strokes that won't disrupt his relaxed state.

1. Begin by standing at your partner's head, with both hands on his upper back in a contact hold. (You can kneel at his head if you're using a mat on the floor.)

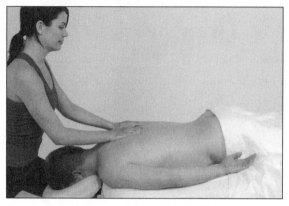

Begin with a contact hold.

2. Next, do some *bilateral* effleurage. Without picking up your hands, glide both hands down your partner's back all the way to his waist. Then pull your hands up his back, going all the way around his shoulders, toward his neck in front of his shoulders, and then up the back of his neck.

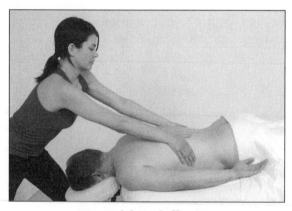

Move to bilateral effleurage.

3. This stroke connects all the parts of the back and shoulders and has a delightful flowing and cohesive feel to it. Perform at least four to six of these strokes.

Definition

When you do something on both sides of your partner at the same time, this is referred to as **bilateral**.

4. On your last stroke down to the waist, press his sacrum toward his feet and hold your hands there for a few breaths, stretching out his lower back. This compression is not a downward pressure toward the front of the body, but rather a lengthening of the back.

5. Standing or sitting at your partner's hip and facing toward his head, place one hand near his waist and make a short effleurage stroke a few inches up his back. Follow your first hand with your other hand, lifting your first hand before your other hand reaches it. Keep repeating this stroke, gradually working your way all the way up to his shoulder in a smooth, alternating hand flow.

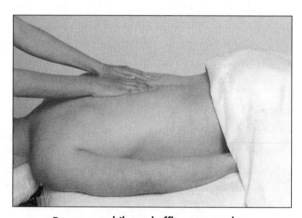

Progress to bilateral effleurage strokes.

6. When you reach his shoulder, move directly into six or eight large circles around his shoulder blade (scapula) as a continuation of the pushing strokes. One set of this flowing sequence is adequate.

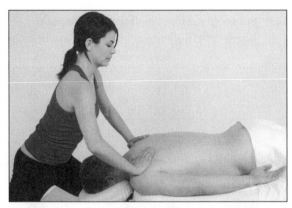

Hands come around the shoulders when returning up from the waist.

7. Moving to his side, place one hand just to your side of his spine, and perform a short effleurage stroke away from you on the opposite side of his spine with your other hand. One hand pins the muscles on the side near you while the other stretches the muscles on the other side of his back.

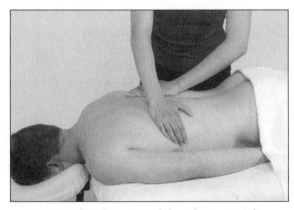

Use one hand to pin and the other to stretch.

8. Continue to pin and stretch out to the side all the way up to his shoulders. You can move back down to his waist again if he seems to be enjoying it or if you feel a lot of tension in the long muscles along his spine.

Getting to the Shoulders and Hips

Petrissage of the shoulders comes next. It's easy to move from the pin and stretch motions into applying petrissage on your partner's shoulders.

1. With the heels of your hand on his upper shoulders and your fingers in front, bring the heels of your hands toward your fingers, squeezing and kneading his shoulder muscles. You may also keep the heels of your hands in place and bring your fingers back toward them as a variation of this stroke. Ask your partner which variation feels better to him. Do at least 8 to 10 of these bilateral strokes.

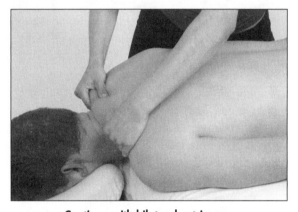

Continue with bilateral petrissage.

Press Here

Alternately, you can apply petrissage to his shoulders unilaterally, that is, one shoulder at a time: massage the shoulder closest to you, lifting and squeezing his shoulder muscles in one palm and then the other, feeding the muscles from one palm to the other at least 10 times. Be sure to keep your full palm on his muscles, as applying this stroke with your fingers will feel uncomfortably "pinchy."

2. Standing near his shoulder, use your closer hand to perform circular friction strokes around the entire border of his closer scapula (shoulder blade). These strokes are little circles with your fingers or thumbs, depending on which part of the scapula you're exploring and which keeps your wrist in a more neutral position.

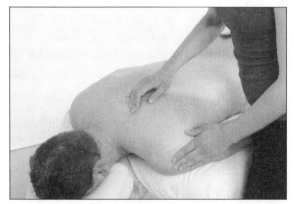

Next come circular friction strokes around the scapula.

3. Continue in an area until you get a good feel for the muscles and underlying bone, and then follow the edge of the bone and explore further. Move to the hip area and do the same kind of circular friction along the crest of the opposite hip. (Massaging on the opposite side of his body keeps you from hyper-extending your wrist as you would if you performed the circular friction on the side closest to you.) It's usually easier to locate the hip (*ilium*) if you palpate for it toward the front of his body. Repeat on the other side.

4. Still standing at your partner's side near his hip, and facing toward his head, start with your hands on each side of the spine close to his hips. Slide your hands up, outward, and then back down and in toward his spine, making a heart shape with your hands. Move your hands up toward his head a few inches and repeat. Keep applying these heart-shaped strokes until you get all the way up to his shoulders; this should

take four or five "hearts." One set of hearts of effleurage is sufficient.

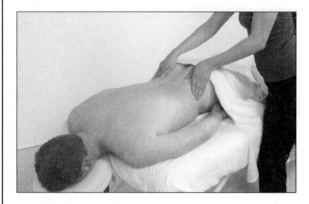

Time for hearts of effleurage.

✋ Back Off _____

Always avoid putting pressure on the spinous processes of the vertebrae.

5. Standing or sitting again at his head, and using one hand on each side of his spine, work up and down his back with whichever forms of tapotement he enjoys: beating, hacking, slapping, tapping, or cupping. Remember to keep your wrists loose and floppy as you apply tapotement, both for your partner's comfort and for the comfort of your wrists, and only apply this percussive stroke for a minute or so.

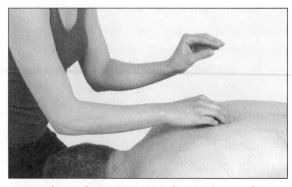

Remember to keep your wrists loose when performing tapotement.

6. Connect your partner's whole back by repeating effleurage just as you did at the beginning of the back sequence.

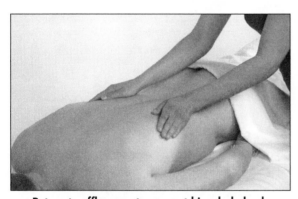

Return to effleurage to connect his whole back.

7. End this back massage with a contact hold on his upper back for three to five breaths.

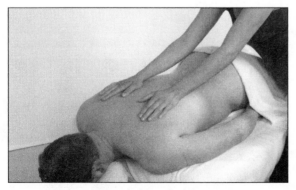

Another contact hold ends this sequence.

Back Massage Tips and Variations

If your partner has discomfort in his lower back when lying prone (face down), place a pillow under his abdomen and chest to flatten the curve of his lower back and make the position more comfortable.

The prone position often causes more arch in the back with large-breasted women, too, putting strain on the back. In this case, place the pillow between her breasts and her lower abdomen to flatten out the lower back curve. Another option is to avoid the prone position entirely and massage your partner in a side-lying position.

Back massage can also be performed with your partner seated. (See Chapters 6 and 7 for more about seated massage.)

The Least You Need to Know

- ◆ The back is well suited to long strokes along each side of the spine.
- ◆ Most back massage is done with your partner lying prone, but it can also be done with your partner lying on his side or even seated.
- ◆ Pinning with one hand and stretching with the other is a particularly useful stroke to use on the back.

In This Chapter

- The identity crisis of the hips
- Working with sensitivity on the hips
- Positions for hip massage
- Vi-i-i-i-bra-a-a-a-tion is gr-r-r-r-reat

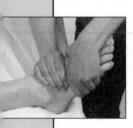
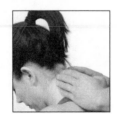
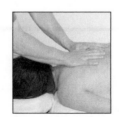
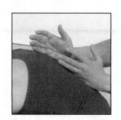
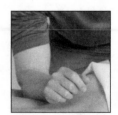
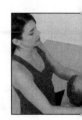

Chapter 12

The Hips

When people think of the hips, many different parts of anatomy come to mind. It's enough to give the hips an identity crisis! Let's set the record straight before we go any further.

Technically, the hip is the joint where the long leg bone (the femur) fits into the socket of the pelvis. But in massage, generally when we speak of hips we also include the area that includes the iliac crest, and the gluteal muscles. This area spans much of the back side of the body from the tops of your legs to your waistline. This much-maligned area of the body is critical for walking, running, climbing, all sports, getting into and out of chairs, and protecting the pelvis from whatever hard surface we sit on.

Using Sensitivity When Massaging the Hips

Receiving good gluteal massage is just as wonderful as receiving massage in other areas, and perhaps more so, as often this area gets little touch attention. But many of us aren't fond of this area of the body, and having someone massage this area might make some people very uncomfortable.

Plus, like the chest and abdominal areas, some people may hold emotions in the gluteal/hip area. Some people associate touch to the buttock area with spankings or whippings as a child, or even sexual or physical abuse. By massaging this area, you could possibly bring up negative memories or emotions—the opposite of the relaxation and enjoyment a massage is supposed to bring.

Back Off _____

For a variety of personal reasons, some people cannot even consider having the gluteal area touched, so find out ahead of time how your partner feels about the area. It's best to ask while your partner is still dressed and upright and in a more comfortable position to say "no" if that's her preference, rather than when she's face down under a drape.

Hip Massage: Getting Started

With some care and sensitivity, you can help your partner enjoy a good hip massage, if that's what she wants. Here's how:

1. When you've cleared gluteal/hip massage with your receiver, begin by standing or kneeling beside her hip as she lies in the prone position. Reach across to her other buttock and hip, applying petrissage for 30 seconds to a minute to the opposite "cheek" to warm it up, staying well away from the gluteal cleavage. (See draping guidelines in Chapter 2.)

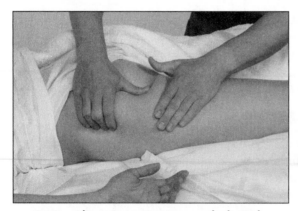

Begin with petrissage to warm up the buttock.

2. In the same position, apply circular friction all around the point of her hip on the other side of her body for a minute.

This enables your wrists to be in a neutral position while working on this area. Many muscles attach at this flattened point, which is about 1×2-inches in size. You might feel them like spokes radiating up, back, and down from the hip.

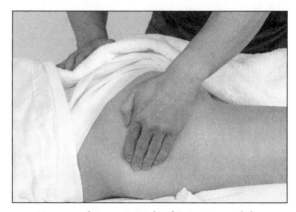

Next, apply some circular friction around the hip joint.

3. If you bring your hands to the center of her back, just below her waist, you'll find the sacrum. This is a roughly triangular bony area about the size of your partner's hand. It feels wonderful to your partner to have vigorous circular friction and vibration all over this bony area for about 20 to 30 seconds. Note this is one of the few times when you'll apply vigorous strokes directly onto a bone.

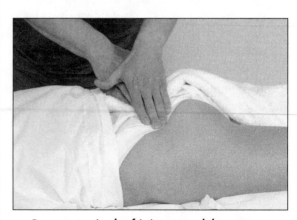

Progress to circular friction around the sacrum.

4. Moving out from the sacrum to the side on the bony ridge (the iliac crest), apply circular friction along the iliac crest, which arches from the sacrum to her side, just below the waistline. Repeat on the other side.

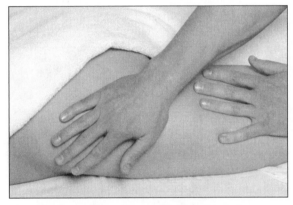

Perform effleurage on the gluteal muscles.

As with the back (see Chapter 11), if your receiver has had any lower back surgery, be very cautious about massaging the hip area.

Back Off

If your partner has pain, numbness, or tingling from the hip and radiating down her leg, it might be best to have her consult her medical professional before receiving massage to this area.

Alternative Petrissage of the Hip Area

An alternative to working with your partner in the prone (face down) position is to massage her as she lies on her side, with a pillow under her head, a pillow between her knees and ankles, and a "huggy" pillow in front of her body.

At Your Fingertips

The pillow under your partner's head in the side-lying position should support her head in such a way that her neck remains in alignment with her spine.

1. Sitting or standing behind her by her hip, apply petrissage to the whole hip and buttock area you have access to for about 30 seconds to 1 minute. Finding the *greater trochanter* and applying circular friction is easier with your partner lying on her side as well.

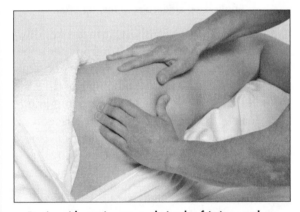

Begin with petrissage and circular friction strokes.

Definition

The large bone you can feel on the side of your partner's hip is the top end of the upper leg bone, known as the *femur*. The rounded protrusion you feel is called the **greater trochanter**.

2. Then apply four or five short, firm effleurage strokes from the edge of her sacrum out to her greater trochanter. You'll probably find some tender areas. You can simply stop and hold your hand firmly on these areas, and many will gradually

"melt." Make several strokes, gliding from her sacrum to hip, until you feel the area has smoothed out.

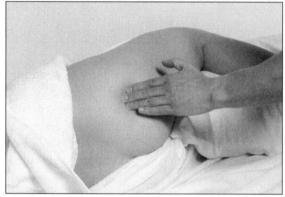

Apply deep effleurage to the hip area.

3. Apply 5 to 10 very short, firm strokes down toward your partner's thigh from her upper hip area, going right over the greater trochanter to the upper and outer thigh. This helps release tension held in her hip joint, making it feel like there's more space in the joint. These strokes should go no more than an inch or 2 below the hip joint.

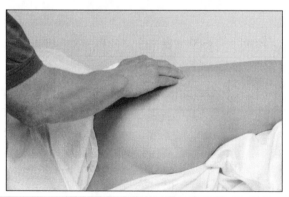

Work with short, deep strokes.

4. Those who believe, usually incorrectly, that their bottoms are too fat probably won't enjoy vibration on their gluteal muscles, but for those who are comfortable with it, it is a wonderfully loosening experience. Placing your palm flat on the gluteal area, create a waving motion with your hand so you can see a ripple effect through the whole area and possibly radiating into her back and thigh. Do this for about 20 seconds.

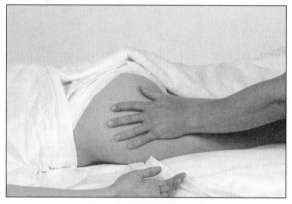

Vibration of the hip area feels great if your receiver is comfortable with the idea.

5. Finish with a contact hold for a few of your partner's breaths.

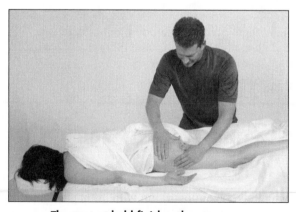

The contact hold finishes the sequence.

The Least You Need to Know

- ◆ People are usually more sensitive about their hips than many other parts of their body.
- ◆ Because of possible emotional involvement, great care is needed when working on the hips.
- ◆ You can massage the hip area with your partner either prone or lying on her side.

In This Chapter

- ◆ What is range of motion?

- ◆ Encouraging more freedom of movement

- ◆ Specific range of motion techniques for different body areas

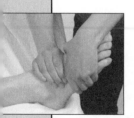
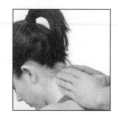
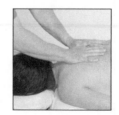
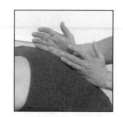
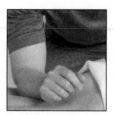
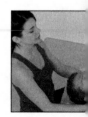

Range of Motion

"Range of motion" refers to techniques that use stretch and other movements to enhance and extend how far the limbs and other areas of the body extend their normal comfortable range limits. Range of motion often is limited in people who do not follow a very regular practice of stretching or yoga. Even those who do stretch regularly often may benefit from passive stretching, which is having someone else perform the movements that extend the available stretch for limbs and other areas of the body. That's where this chapter comes in.

Range of Motion Precautions

When working with someone's range of motion or applying passive stretches, be sure to follow these guidelines:

◆ Support joints as you move your partner's limb.

◆ Be sure to not hyperextend, or push the joint into too much of a stretch at any time.

◆ Make the movements very slowly and very conservatively. If you move a limb too fast you may "blow through" or pass an acceptable amount of stretch. This can cause discomfort, guarding by the person to protect the area, or injury in the worst case. As you continue to move the limb, you may be able to slowly and gently increase the amount of stretch.

At Your Fingertips

Communication is critical in doing all massage, but it is especially important in working with range of motion. It's imperative that your partner understands that she must communicate to you if any movement even approaches feeling like it's too much. Also, watch her face for any sign of discomfort as you apply movement and stretches.

◆ End points are the places where you feel that the area does not want to move any more. To sense end points, you must be fully focused on what you're doing and be exquisitely sensitive to the slowing of motion as you approach the limit. If there's any question in your mind about whether you can feel the end points, don't attempt to use this technique.

Range of motion is best applied at the end of massage to each area of the body. Muscles are more pliable then, and joints move more freely after the area is warmed up with effleurage and petrissage.

Be advised that range of motion work is not for everyone. Some people are unable to give their limbs up to the passive movements and will either hold the area or try to take over the movement on their own. This simply doesn't work. You have two options: either you can ask your partner to allow the limb to be heavy and concentrate on her breathing, or you can go on to other massage techniques. Never make a receiver feel she is wrong because she has difficulty letting go and allowing you to perform passive movements with her body.

Arms and Hands: Wrist Flexion/Extension

The following range of motion techniques are done with your partner relaxing in the supine (face up) position.

1. After warming up her arm with effleurage and petrissage, lift her hand off the table or mat, leaving her elbow in place.

2. As you raise her hand with one of your hands on the pinky side and the other on the thumb side, flex her wrist so her palm is gently pressed toward her inner wrist.

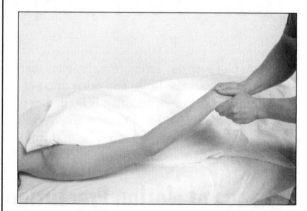

Flex your partner's wrist up and down several times.

3. Bring her hand back down toward the table surface, extending her wrist gently toward the back of her arm (the opposite direction from the wrist flexion you just did) so the underside of her wrist moves more closely to the table than her fingers.

4. Repeat two to four times.

Shoulders: Arm-Over

After you've completed massaging her arm and shoulder …

1. Slide one hand under the shoulder (scapula) as you use your other hand to bring her arm across her chest. Find the edge of the scapula closest to her spine, and curl your fingers there against the edge of the shoulder blade closest to the spine.

2. With your other hand, gently rock the elbow away from you. You'll feel the movement of the scapula with your fingers curled at its edge.

3. Gradually, as the muscles of her upper back relax, you'll notice that her arm will rock a little farther away from you with each press of your hand just above her elbow. The rocking should be at the rate of about 1 rock per 2 seconds, although the rate at which the upper arm comes back toward you after each rock will vary from person to person. You may rock the elbow over at least a dozen times.

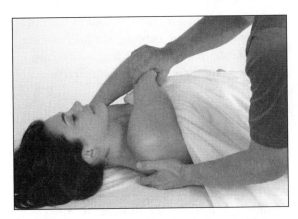

This work stretches both the arm and shoulder.

4. Repeat on the other side after you have massaged that arm, hand, and shoulder.

Hips: Knee-Over Leg Rock

After you've completed massaging her foot, leg, and thigh …

1. Place one hand under her thigh just above her knee and your other hand on the sole of her foot. Lift her thigh slightly as you push her foot toward her buttocks.

2. Place your knee on the mat or table surface just beyond her foot so her foot won't slide toward the end of the table, and slowly push her leg and thigh away from you.

3. Begin to rock her leg gently away from you, keeping your hand on her thigh, near the knee.

4. Perform the leg rocking for about 30 seconds.

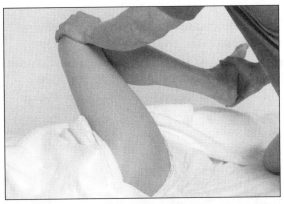

The knee-over leg rock is the first step in range of motion on the leg.

You don't need to pull her leg back toward you—it will come back by itself, and the rate at which her leg returns will determine the rhythm of the rocking. Don't let her leg come all the way back toward you, but keep a slight pressure away from you, even as her leg rebounds back toward you. Gradually, her leg will move freely farther across her other leg than when you started the rocking. You can move your hand up and down her thigh as you rock her leg, rather than leaving your hand in one position on her leg. You can also use your other hand at her hip to intensify the rocking movement of her leg and thigh.

Legs: Helicopter

Following the opening of the hips with the knee-over ...

1. Lift her foot, using your hand on the sole of her foot, at the same level as her knee. Keep enough pressure on her foot in the direction of her head so her leg stays up just from the flexion of her hip toward her chest.

2. Using your hand at her knee to steer the movement, make 8 or 10 slow and gentle circles with her knee and lower leg. These circles will gradually increase in size as her hip and leg loosens up.

3. Maintain sensitivity to feel when you're close to the end points of her stretch. Move her leg slowly, and don't try to push past end points. At the same time, you want the circles to be large enough that she feels the stretch.

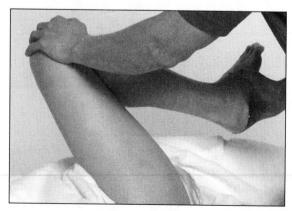

Make your circles big enough so she can feel the stretch, but don't exceed her limits.

Feet and Ankles

Following a warm-up of effleurage and petrissage of the foot and ankle area, you can perform a variety of movements on your partner's foot to loosen up her ankle:

1. Cupping her heel in your hand, with your arm against the sole of her foot, lean toward her head until you feel the stretch.

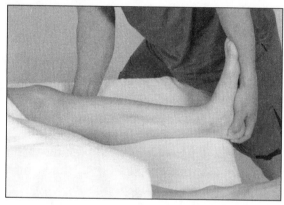

Lean toward your partner's head until you feel the stretch.

2. Release and repeat a couple more times.

3. Then hold your partner's foot in both of your hands, one cupping her heel and the other on the ball of her foot, and rotate her ankle three times in each direction.

Shoulders

We now switch to range of motion techniques applied while your partner is in the side-lying position, which gives you the best access to the shoulders, and allows the shoulder to rotate freely.

1. Standing at her back, or sitting on the table behind her, reach under her upper arm and cup the front of her shoulder (deltoid) with that hand. Place your other hand on her scapula.

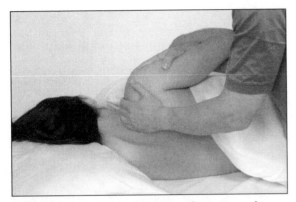

This is how you begin the range of motion work on the shoulders.

2. In a smooth, coordinated circular movement, rotate her shoulder up toward her ear, back toward you, and then down toward her hip.

3. Repeat this motion three to five times.

You can repeat the movement, rotating her shoulder in the opposite direction to see which she prefers, although this direction has the benefit of opening the chest muscles more effectively. You may stop the motion at any point where you feel some resistance to the motion and ask her to breathe into the area, relaxing muscles and softening any resistance.

Arms and Shoulders: Shoulder Broadening

After you've massaged your partner's back, hips, and shoulders, and with your partner in the prone position …

1. Stand at the side of the table and grasp her arm a couple inches above her elbow.

2. Taking her arm in one or both hands, lean back, away from the table so you're broadening her shoulder.

3. Swing her lower arm back and forth about eight times, using your whole body to transmit the swinging motion into her arm and shoulder.

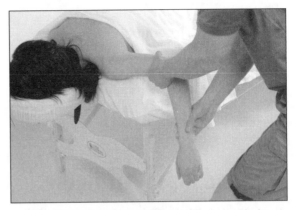

Begin the arm and shoulder broadening with this arm-swinging work.

4. At the end of the arm, hand, and shoulder sequence on that side of the body, bring your partner's whole arm and hand onto the table. Grasp her wrist and her upper arm just above the elbow.

5. Keeping her wrist and elbow up off the table, move her lower arm in circles away from you (over her back), up toward her head, and then back toward you.

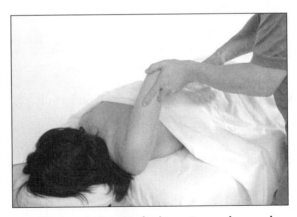

Moving the arm is great for loosening up the muscles in the arm and extending its range of motion.

6. Move slowly and sensitively through at least six full rotations, keeping the wrist almost at the level of the elbow.

7. Repeat on the other arm after massaging that arm, hand, and shoulder.

At Your Fingertips

You can rotate her arm and shoulder in the opposite direction as well, or move from one direction of rotation to the other to confuse a receiver who is trying to help by moving her arm for you.

Legs and Hips: Calf Jiggle

After you've warmed up the back of your partner's leg and hip on one side …

1. Lift up her foot until her lower leg is perpendicular to the table.

2. Hold her big toe and the ball of her foot near the big toe so your palm is facing upward and your thumb is facing you.

3. Using an up-and-down motion that comes from your legs, flick her heel away from you rhythmically. Her calf will jiggle as you transfer the movement from your body through her foot to her leg.

4. You may move the foot farther away or closer to you as you apply the flicking movements for about 30 seconds.

This loosens the calf muscles wonderfully.

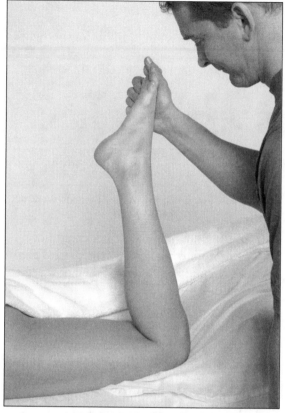

This range-of-motion exercise relaxes and loosens the calf muscles.

The Least You Need to Know

◆ Most people don't use their limbs to their full capacity because they don't stretch their muscles to their full extent.

◆ Range of motion work can increase how far people can flex or extend their limbs and other body parts.

◆ Range of motion can be effective if your partner is passive and able to relax.

In This Part

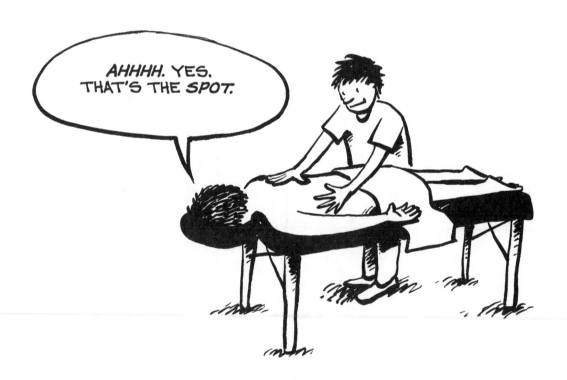

Massage Combinations for Specific Problems

Massage can be used to help with a wide variety of conditions that plague us and make our lives less fulfilling than they ought to be. Part 3 deals with those conditions and how best to reduce or eliminate the problems they cause. The purpose of this part is not to turn you into a medical professional, but to give you the basic knowledge needed to help people with specific problems. You might be able to help your partner live a more fulfilling life with reduced pain and problems.

A note, though: if problems are severe or persistent; related to a recent injury or surgery; or are accompanied by fever, redness, swelling, and significant dysfunction, they should be evaluated by a health-care practitioner.

In This Chapter

- ◆ Using massage to alleviate TMJ problems
- ◆ Massaging away headaches
- ◆ Easing sinus congestion problems

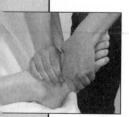 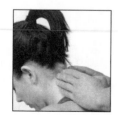 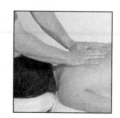 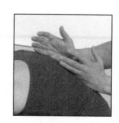 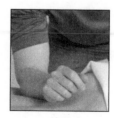 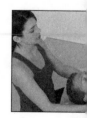

Chapter 14

Head and Neck Conditions

Massage works very well on head and neck problems. The conditions we explore in this chapter—TMJ problems, headaches, neck pain, and sinus problems—can overlap or contribute to each other, so often it's beneficial to address all the conditions during a massage, especially if a headache is your partner's primary discomfort.

Temporomandibular Joint Discomfort

The temporomandibular joint (TMJ) is between your lower jaw and your skull, just in front of your ear. Put your fingers on the side of your face and open and close your jaw, and you'll feel the outward motion at this joint as your jaw opens. Clicking or popping of the jaw; jaw locking; or head, neck, face, tooth, and jaw pain can all be associated with wear and tear on a small disc of connective tissue that cushions the TM joint. These kinds of discomfort and dysfunction can be brought about by misaligned teeth, gum chewing, teeth grinding, dental procedures, and other activities that tax the jaw, especially stress.

The head, face, neck, and shoulder areas will ordinarily be tight if someone is experiencing TMJ issues, as they tend to tighten up all the muscles in the area to "guard" the areas of pain. Plus, pain from TMJ often spills over into the head, face, and neck. If stress is the precipitating factor in setting off TMJ problems, there's perhaps nothing better than a relaxing massage in the entire area—or better yet, the entire body. Most of the forceful actions we perform with our jaw muscles are closing actions, like biting down on something. Therefore, the massage strokes we use will be aimed at creating space and lengthening the major chewing muscles, the *masseter* and *temporalis* muscles.

1. With your partner supine, apply relaxing massage to the whole head, face, neck, and shoulder area.

2. After you've completed the general relaxing massage techniques, bring your fingers to the sides of your partner's face near the angle of his jaw bone and apply anywhere from 10 to 30 firm downward strokes from his cheekbone to his mandible (jaw bone).

3. Staying in the same area of the side of the lower face, apply circular friction for 10 to 20 seconds, feeling for any remaining areas of tension.

Press Here

These firm downward strokes are called *stripping strokes* because they're a short stroke in one direction only. This helps you create length in the muscle.

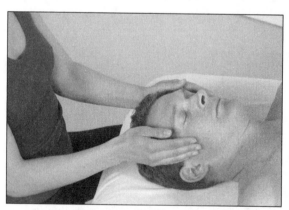

Apply circular friction to the sides of the face and jaw.

If during either stripping or circular friction you feel like he's "fighting" you—not allowing his jaw to become slack and relaxed—you might want to suggest that he place the edge of his tongue between his back teeth on one side. This will stop him from tensing his jaw as you try to help loosen it. Often, individuals with TMJ problems have forgotten how to allow their jaws to relax. Massage can help them find that comfort again, but like any habit, it can be a challenge to break.

Headaches

There are numerous kinds of headaches, but one thing they all have in common is tension. Even if a headache has begun as a result of sinus congestion or barometric pressure affecting the sinuses, caffeine withdrawal, TMJ, allergies, or migraine circulatory problems, once the pain begins, almost all headache sufferers "guard" the area by tensing the face, scalp, neck, and shoulder muscles. Tension headaches arise primarily from the effects of tension and stress in these areas.

As with TMJ, the place to begin is with a relaxing head, face, neck, and shoulder massage. Or better yet, offer a full-body massage to assist the headache sufferer in relaxing all her muscles and especially those in and near her head.

After you've completed general relaxing massage of the area …

1. Find the slight indentation just in front of her ear, where the top of her ear joins her face. Gently hold your index fingers in this small indentation on both sides of her face for about 30 seconds.

2. Apply firm slow circles at her temples for another 30 seconds.

3. Perform firm, slow circular friction across her occipital ridge (base of the skull) and up and down each side of the spine on her neck.

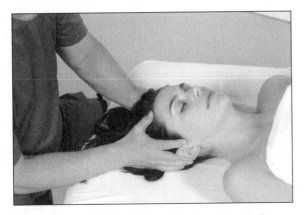

Pressure on this point can relieve some headaches.

4. Every now and then, simply stop, with your hands resting on her forehead in a contact hold, and coordinate your breath with hers. This technique, while simple, is comforting and, in the case of a bad headache, can be more tolerable than a lot of movement.

Although we have indicated the amount of time to spend on an area or how many particular strokes, that is a very general guideline to get you started. If your partner has a lot of tension in an area apply the stroke for a longer period of time or for more repetitions. The very essence of massage is that you do not follow a set pattern for a specific period of time, but rather allow your partner's body to "speak" to you about what is needed during the particular massage session. All the suggested sequences in this book can be changed in terms of the order and duration of the segments depending on your partner's needs. If massage is a dance, your partner leads; to dance well you need to pay attention to her body's signals to you.

Sinus Congestion

Acupressure is extremely effective in relieving sinus congestion, after you have warmed up the area with effleurage and circular friction. The amount of force you exert in pressure-point massage is small, but calm and patient.

At Your Fingertips

Be sure to warm up your partner's face with effleurage and friction before using pressure on specific points.

1. Start by placing the pads of your thumbs on your partner's nose, specifically on the nasal bones, which are about ¼-inch long below the bridge of the nose.

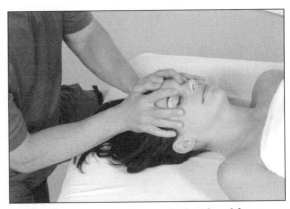

Pressure on certain points on the head and face can help ease sinus congestion.

2. Your fingers will be pointed up in almost a prayer position while you apply gentle pressure on the nasal bones for about 30 seconds, each thumb pressing toward your other thumb.

3. Work your way from the point where the crease above her nostril joins her cheek, pressing there for about a few seconds,

and then along the base of her cheekbone, stopping and holding pressure points for several seconds wherever you sense them.

4. Be sure to press directly below the pupil of her eye along the cheekbone for several seconds.

At Your Fingertips

The pressure on all these points is not straight in, but angled upward, as if your fingers are pointing toward the crown of her head.

5. End with the headache point indentation where her ear joins her face for another 30 seconds. Don't angle up on this point, but apply the gentle pressure straight in.

In general, stimulating the acupressure points for sinus congestion opens the sinuses and releases pressure anywhere from immediately following the massage to 20 or 30 minutes after your partner is upright again and off the table.

Back Off

For anyone who is experiencing sinus congestion, sinus headache, or allergies that affect the sinuses, the prone position for massage is not recommended. It will just make their noses and sinuses more stuffy.

The Least You Need to Know

◆ TMJ problems can feel miserable. Massage is one way to lessen the pain.

◆ Headaches plague us all from time to time, and massage can provide relief for many.

◆ Although sinus trouble can't be cured with massage, it can bring some relief from the discomfort.

In This Chapter

- ◆ Is massage right for a specific back problem?
- ◆ Easing muscle spasms
- ◆ Aiding posture problems

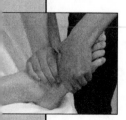
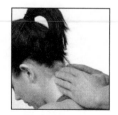
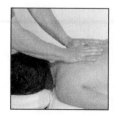
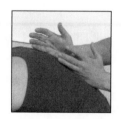
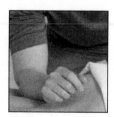
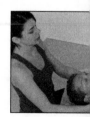

Chapter 15

Back Complaints

A lot more goes on with your back than you may be aware of on a regular basis. You don't see your own back (unless you employ a mirror or two), and many people seldom think much about their backs unless it itches or hurts. Like the rest of your body, the back thrives on movement. Maintaining a rigid or still posture, especially in a seated or standing position, for long periods of time will make almost anyone's back hurt. Standing at a counter or cash register or sitting at a computer for 8 hours a day is probably harder on your back than doing heavier work.

The best way to deal with back pain is to avoid it in the first place by establishing and maintaining a regular schedule of stretching and strengthening exercises. Even the strongest and most flexible back is vulnerable to pain and stiffness from time to time, regardless of how careful you are, or how much your exercise program. Massage can help.

When Massage Is Appropriate—and When It Isn't

If back pain comes on within 48 hours of unaccustomed activity, such as sports or mowing the grass for the first time in the spring, chances are good it's simply overuse and perhaps muscle spasm. But self-diagnosis is tricky, and if there is any electrical-shock sort of sensation or loss of feeling in an area, such as down a leg, it's probably best to go see your chiropractor or physician.

Many doctors will tell you frightening things when you visit them about back pain. You're likely to hear such phrases as "degenerative disc disease," "arthritic changes to the spine," and "narrowed disc spaces," if you're over 40.

Well, welcome to life on a planet with gravity! We all tend to develop narrowed disc spaces as we age, and these may be considered a—*gasp!*—degenerative condition. More often than not, these conditions are not associated with pain; those who have narrowed disc spaces may or may not have discomfort. The same thing is true with bulging, herniated (sometimes called "slipped") discs. More often the pain you feel is muscle spasm, because the muscles are seeking to protect an area where there are changes in the bony architecture. Numbness is almost always worse news than pain. Pain will unrelentingly direct you toward what makes it worse or better. If you listen to what your body is telling you, often that will be all you need to do to decrease your discomfort. Numbness is most often a signal that a spinal nerve is indeed being pinched and is a sign to go to your doctor or chiropractor.

Pain that doesn't resolve quickly is another signal to head in your doctor's direction and to ask your physician or chiropractor to recommend a massage therapist and prescribe massage therapy. In some areas of the country, health insurance covers professional massage—which, in the case of significant back or neck problems, is a very good idea. And even if your insurance won't cover treatment, if you have a prescription for massage therapy, you can itemize it as a medical tax deduction. Serious back and neck injuries are nothing for the amateur to massage.

Press Here

Back pain is one of the biggest contributors to lost time from work.

But supposing you're just a little sore and you have a pretty good idea of the activity that set off the pain. That's a good time to get massage, to have a hot shower, and to cut back on whatever activity resulted in back pain.

Muscle Spasms

A muscle spasm is ordinarily a pain that "grabs" you when you move in a certain way. The following massage techniques may help for muscle spasm and focuses on the most common area for such spasms: the lower back, or directly behind the waist. Of course, you can target other areas of the back using the same basic methods.

At Your Fingertips

It may be helpful to place a pillow under the prone receiver from his chest to his groin area. This puts greater stretch into the lower back muscles when a muscle spasm is occurring. Try it and ask your partner how it feels compared with lying flat on the table. Do not forget to place a pillow under your partner's lower legs when your partner is in the prone position as well.

1. If you have a heat pack, rest it on the area of his muscle spasm for 10 minutes before you start the massage.

2. Start with your partner in the prone position, and perform a contact hold on his shoulders.

3. Warm up his whole back with effleurage, standing at the head of the table and moving your hands from his shoulders all the way down to his hips, and back up and around his shoulders.

4. Do this at least six times, each time leaning into the stroke a little more, increasing the pressure. Be sure to be sensitive and focused, searching for any area that feels, dense, tight, and contracted as you perform the strokes. This will be the area of the spasm.

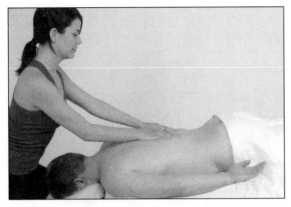

Apply effleurage to the back.

5. Feel for other problem areas elsewhere on his back. These may well contribute to the spasm that is causing his discomfort.

6. On the last effleurage stroke, hold your palms on his sacrum and apply pressure, not straight down but toward his feet, for about 10 seconds. Then, bring your hands back up and around his shoulders.

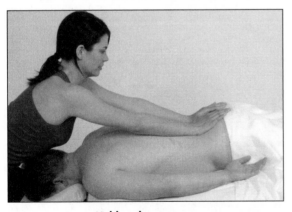

Hold at the sacrum.

7. Stand by the side of the table and apply petrissage to the opposite side of his back, lifting and squeezing the muscles vigorously, increasing blood flow to the area for a couple minutes.

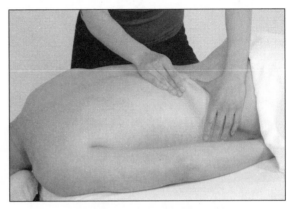

Apply petrissage to the back.

8. After you've thoroughly applied petrissage to that side of his back, place one hand just to the side of his spine near you, and make a stroke with your other hand and forearm on the opposite side of his spine, pushing over and down his side. (This stroke is called pin and stretch because you're stabilizing the flesh on one side of the spine as you stretch the muscles on the opposite side away from the spine.)

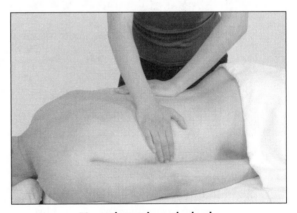

Pin and stretch on the back.

9. Start at his waist and make two strokes in each hand position as you move gradually all the way up to his shoulder blades.

10. Then perform an alternating hand-pushing stroke up the near side of his back, one hand "chasing" the other hand until you are all the way up to his shoulder.

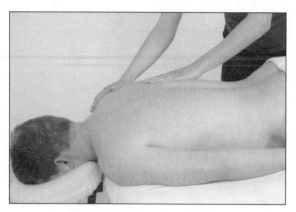

Alternate hand-pushing stroke.

11. At his shoulder, apply petrissage on his near shoulder, feeding the tissue from one hand to the other several times before moving to the other side of the table, and repeat these four sets of strokes from the other side.

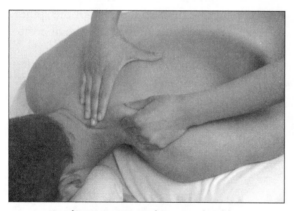

Apply petrissage on his near shoulder.

12. Standing at the side of the table at his hip, begin to explore, or palpate, the area just above his hip bone (iliac crest). Because you've already warmed up this area with effleurage and petrissage, you can explore pretty deeply to feel for taut "ropey bands" or areas that feel congested and tight.

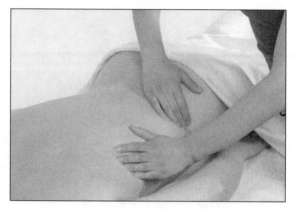

Palpation of the iliac crest.

13. Perform small back-and-forth or circular friction all along his iliac crest on the side near you for about 3 minutes. Repeat on the other side of his back.

14. Next, still standing at his hip, apply effleurage up his back and then back down to his hips. About eight of these strokes will smooth out the area you were palpating and further warm up the back muscles.

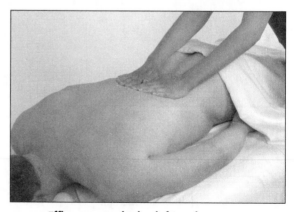

Effleurage up the back from the sacrum.

15. Return to the head of the table and perform tapotement if he can relax into the percussive motions. Be sure to check with him about whether tapotement feels good to his back muscles.

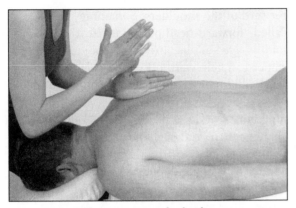

Tapotement on the back.

If you don't have a massage table, you can still perform this back massage. Simply have your partner lie on a mat on the floor. You can then kneel next to him.

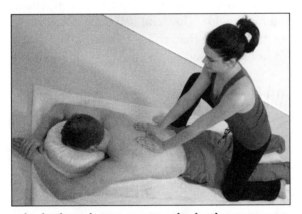

This back-work sequence can also be done on a mat on the floor.

Posture Problems

People display a wide variety of postural abnormalities, and massage can help ease the resulting discomforts, regardless of whether the conditions are temporary or permanent. We will look at three of the most common postural abnormalities:

- Scoliosis
- Lordosis
- Kyphosis

Scoliosis

Scoliosis is a curvature of the spine from side to side and is usually most evident in the mid-back area. Once the spine has assumed the curve in adulthood, it usually won't change very much. Performing the kind of massage listed in Chapters 11 and 12 works well for the discomforts associated with scoliosis because it frequently affects the hips as well as the back. You may also approach work on the back of a receiver who has scoliosis as you would in the earlier "Muscle Spasms" section.

Frequently, the side of the back that the spine curves toward is in some degree of spasm all the time. You'll notice the muscles on that side of the person's back are frequently more developed and rise higher than those on the other side of the back. All back massage may be modified so you spend more time on the side of your partner's back that has the tighter muscles.

Lordosis

Lordosis is an abnormally extreme curve in the lower back, and it frequently can be changed with strengthening exercises and attention to posture, even in adulthood. The muscles in the person's lower back will be tight and may be prone to spasms, so we recommend approaching massage in the same way you would for a lower back spasm.

If you perform a full-body massage on a person with lordosis, it's especially important not to forget the pillow under the knees and lower thighs when he's in the supine position, as bolstering in this way takes the strain off the lower back and enables it to flatten against the table surface.

Lordosis is frequently accompanied by lower-back pain. In Chapter 19, we discuss acupressure points and techniques that can assist with lower back discomfort. All the indentations in the sacrum (the bone between the lower back and the tailbone) are useful pressure points for lower back pain, as are points at the back of the waistline two finger-widths and four finger-widths out from the spine. This group of points was named the Sea of Vitality by the ancient Chinese. In both of these cases, holding points in the areas from 1 to 3 minutes can have striking results.

Press Here

If the person with lordosis is a large-breasted woman, put a pillow under her from just below her breasts to her groin area when she is in the prone position, or she will be lying on the table with her back in precisely the arched position that's causing her problems. The pillow under her torso helps lengthen and straighten her spine, and you might be able to help her relax those muscles that have been chronically shortened.

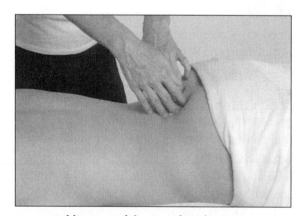

Holding two of the Sea of Vitality points.

Kyphosis

Kyphosis is perhaps the most common postural deviation. Kyphosis is a slumping forward of the shoulders combined with the head stretched forward of the shoulders. Sometimes this is called "forward-head position." In young to middle-aged adults, attention to a more upright stance can help ward off kyphosis later in life. With older people, especially women over 60 years of age, kyphosis can be a result of thinning bones, and the posture is unlikely to change much. Today, many people contribute to their kyphosis by sitting slumped for hours on end in front of a computer. A proper chair and correct keyboard and monitor height can help a lot, as can massage.

Massage is very effective in relieving the aches, pains, and tightness associated with kyphosis. However, the results will be only temporary at best unless the person with this postural problem makes the effort to remember to keep his back and neck straight and lengthened, and his shoulders low and in a normal neutral position, rather than rolled forward following his head.

Back Off

Sitting with your shoulders hunched forward reduces how much air you can inhale. Straightening up and holding your shoulders back and head erect can increase oxygen availability.

Someone with kyphosis and a forward head posture will experience many aches and pains. Even someone who does not exhibit this posture when walking around but who sits at a work station or desk in this position will have similar problems. Most common will be tightness and pain in the upper shoulders, trapezius, rhomboids, and other muscles, which get pulled and stretched as the chest muscles shorten from chronic slumping.

In addition to the sequence earlier in this chapter for back-muscle spasms, it will be useful to add massage around the scapulae to those strokes:

1. When your partner's back is warmed up in the prone position, perform small back-and-forth or circular friction all around the border of his scapulae. This is most easily done from a position standing at the side of the table, once you have completed the warm-up with petrissage, pin and stretch, and effleurage strokes.

2. You might want to take 3 to 5 minutes palpating around the edges of each scapula, as many muscles attach to the shoulder blade, and most of them will be affected by postural problems.

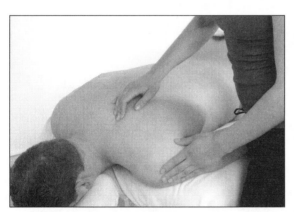

Palpation around the scapula.

3. Follow the relatively deep massage around the scapula with smoothing effleurage.

4. With your partner in the supine position, perform effleurage from the center of his chest out and around his shoulders (deltoid muscles), then toward his spine on the back of his shoulders, and finally up the back of his neck.

5. Repeat this lovely integrating flow of effleurage strokes at least eight times, leaning a bit more heavily into the strokes with each repetition, especially on the upper-chest muscles, which are often

fatigued and sore from the chronic shortening of being rolled forward.

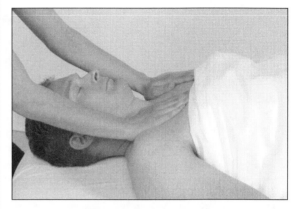

Effleurage of the upper chest.

Press Here _____

A person with head-forward posture both looks and feels as if he is uncertain, shy, and perhaps ashamed about something, "hanging his head." If he changes his posture, he'll begin to both look and feel more confident, and other people will begin to see him differently, treat him differently, and the whole cycle will reinforce his internal and postural change.

Applying massage in these ways can be very helpful in alleviating muscle tightness, soreness, and overstretching. But for continuing relief, strengthening exercises for the upper back muscles are very important in maintaining postural improvement and in preventing further pain.

The Least You Need to Know

◆ Many types of back problems respond well to massage.

◆ Muscle spasms can be very painful, but the muscles often can be relaxed through massage.

◆ Massage can help ease pain caused by postural problems, even later in life.

In This Chapter

- ◆ Massage for tired, aching feet
- ◆ Increasing flexibility with massage
- ◆ Reflexology 101

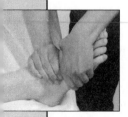 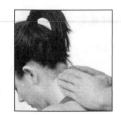 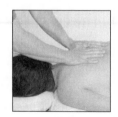 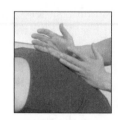 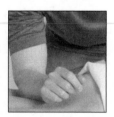 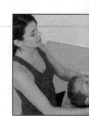

Chapter 16

Oh, My Aching Feet!

Feet are some of the real workhorses in the body, and like many other areas of the body, we don't think much about our feet until they hurt. Our feet support us, carry us around, and help us stay balanced when we're standing.

Most of us have foot problems at one time or another, and knowing how to deal with them can improve quality of life. Foot massage can be a specialty unto itself, but we cover it in enough detail here to provide you with a good basic understanding.

Dealing with Unpleasant Feet

To some, the idea of touching someone's feet is disgusting, and massage therapists are often asked how they can stand to work on people's feet. So here's our take on the issue: there's absolutely nothing wrong with feet. Where would we be (or go!) without them?

True, there's always the possibility of the dreaded "stink foot" in Frank Zappa's words, but in the 5,000 or so massages I have given over the years, I've only had to deal with stinky feet 3 or 4 times. Most people will have the courtesy to come to you with clean tootsies, and if they don't, you can fix that.

Stinky feet or not, your recipient will probably love a nice, refreshing, and relaxing going-over with a hot, soapy washcloth, followed by a warm towel-drying. With this kind of treatment, though, your partner might start making a point of coming for massage with dirty feet! If you don't want to be quite so elaborate, premoistened toilettes or baby wipes do a perfectly adequate job of freshening feet.

Press Here

For those who still have reservations about feet: in those same 5,000 massages, I've probably had 20 cases of raw onion, cigar, or cigarette breath. Talk about challenging! Offering breath mints to these folks helps, but not as much as the actions you can take to freshen feet

If you're hesitant about the cleanliness of feet in general, inexpensive foot spas are available in department stores and drug stores. Have your partner place her feet in the spa while you discuss how she's feeling and the areas she'd like you to concentrate on during her massage. She'll enjoy the hot bubbling water (with disinfectant in it if you prefer) and will already be partly relaxed, with soothed feet, even before her massage begins.

Back Off

If a person has gout, you should definitely avoid even touching her feet. Gout is a condition in which any pressure exerted on the area—usually the big toe—where uric-acid crystals have settled causes a sensation not unlike stepping on broken glass. Pressing on a gouty toe will probably undo any relaxation your partner has gained this far into the massage.

Soothing Tired Feet

Foot spas help clean feet and also relax and soothe tired feet. Microwaveable heat packs, placed on or under the soles of your partner's feet or wrapped around her feet, can be very relaxing, especially if she tends to have cold feet. Hot towels wrapped around her feet have a similar, but not as long-lasting, effect.

Numerous foot creams, most of which contain peppermint oil, have a stimulating and cooling effect on feet that may be tired and hot from having been cooped up in shoes or standing on hot pavement for too long.

And don't forget what we're here for: generally, just massaging feet, as detailed in Chapter 10, dramatically soothes those tired doggies.

Foot Pain

Two conditions cause foot pain for millions of people every year: *plantar fasciitis*, which affects many runners and people who may be carrying some extra weight, and *pes planus*, commonly known as flat feet, which frequently arises as a result of heredity or nonsupportive footwear.

A person with plantar fasciitis often has a lot of pain when her feet hit the floor first thing in the morning, as the fascia has shortened during the night. In extreme cases, just the amount of time someone is on a massage table or mat might be enough to give her extreme pain in the sole of her foot. People with flat feet often experience pain in the plantar surface of their feet as well. In both conditions, the foot problems, if allowed to continue, can cause additional problems in the person's knees, hips, and back.

Press Here

A lot of people have bone spurs on the soles of their feet, near the heel, and it was once thought that these spurs were a source of the pain. But irritation of the fascia on the bottom of the foot (the plantar surface, that is) actually stimulates the growth of bone spurs, and not the other way around.

Fortunately, massage is a good treatment for plantar fasciitis and flat feet, increasing circulation and loosening up connective tissue:

1. Spend at least 3 or 4 minutes warming up your partner's entire foot with effleurage while she's in the supine (face up) position.

2. Apply the milking stroke to her foot. Take the foot that's closest to you in both your hands and perform a series of about 10 strong, short-pulling effleurage strokes first on one side of her foot and then the other. Your strokes should be alternately lengthening each side of her foot.

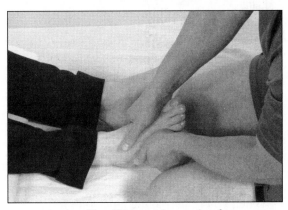

Begin with milking strokes on her foot.

3. Then reverse the action, pushing toward her heel on the arch and the outside of her foot, moving gradually into circles on the front of her ankle.

4. Wring her foot applying the "Indian rub" technique with your thumbs on the middle arch side of the foot, as if you were wringing out a towel. Allow a lot of movement in the foot as you perform the strokes, as it will be good for the range of motion in her ankle and will stimulate circulation.

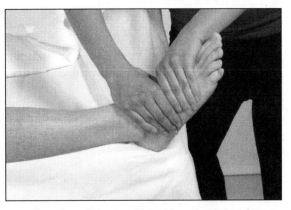

Follow the milking strokes with wringing strokes.

5. After you've revved up the circulation in her foot and warmed the muscles and connective tissue, begin to make long and gradually deeper strokes along the length of the sole of her foot, with one hand on each side of her foot.

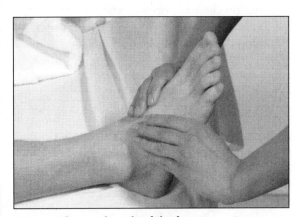

Long strokes on the sole of the foot are an important part of foot massage.

6. You can use the backs of your fingers in a semi-fist to slide firmly from the heel to the ball of her foot with more pressure if that feels better on your hands.

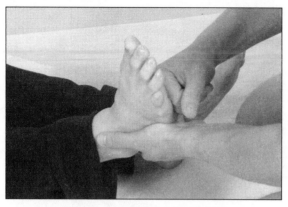

Apply strokes with back of your fingers.

7. Be sure to perform some long effleurage strokes and some petrissage on her whole foot, leg, and thigh area after such specific massage.

8. With your partner prone, you can raise her leg up to vertical, with her thigh resting on the table or mat, and use your forearm or elbow to even more firmly press along the long muscle and connective tissue fibers on the sole of her foot.

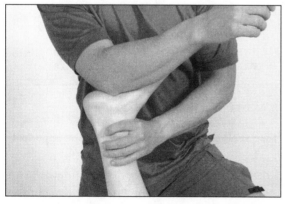

You can use your forearm or elbow to apply pressure to the sole of the foot.

9. When you've completed the specific strokes on her foot, apply petrissage and deep effleurage to her calf muscles. Sometimes tightness in the calf muscles can exert pressure deep in the foot, which contributes to plantar fasciitis and pes planus.

An Introduction to Reflexology

The bottom of each of your feet contain 7,200 nerve endings, and practitioners of reflexology believe the nerves in the feet correspond to different glands, organs, and other parts of the body. Reflexology uses the pressure of fingers, thumbs, or other devices to stimulate points on the foot (and also sometimes the hands and ears) to help relieve stress and tension, unblock nerve impulses, and improve blood supply.

Press Here

It's beyond the scope of this book to certify you in reflexology; someone who is serious about pursuing this form of bodywork should look for a 200-hour program in the field. Check out *The Complete Idiot's Guide to Reflexology*, now in its second edition (Alpha Books, 2006), if you want to learn more.

When you're massaging a person's foot, following the sequence in Chapter 10, concentrate your focus on what you're feeling. In certain areas you'll find little knots or bumps; "crunchies," which are difficult to define, but you'll know them when you feel them; and other areas that feel "boggy," dense, or less energetic than the surrounding tissues. These are areas where you may exert some additional pointed pressure.

As you perform these small compressions on your partner's feet, feel whether the areas you're pressing change in quality as you hold the points for a few seconds. Chances are good you'll feel areas "normalize" and begin to blend in more with the surrounding tissues as you focus pressure and attention there. Be sure to squeeze the toes and palpate the soles of the feet thoroughly if you're interested in exploring the sensations of reflexology.

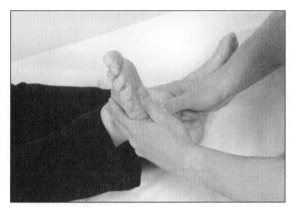

Apply additional pressure on the areas you identify as little knots or bumps.

![At Your Fingertips]
At Your Fingertips

You can enlist numerous other reflex effects in massaging the body besides those of the feet. If, for instance, your partner has a cast on her left leg, massaging the right leg can have a positive effect on circulation and healing of the leg you have no access to.

Increasing Movement and Flexibility in the Feet and Ankles

If your partner has stiffness in her feet, try some range-of-motion actions to help loosen her joints, particularly the ankles:

1. Holding her foot up, so her knee is at a right angle to her thigh in the prone (face down) position, place one hand on her lower leg, just above her ankles.

2. Holding her forefoot in your other hand, gently rotate her foot in circles, changing

the degree to which you flex her ankle as you continue the circles for 9 or 10 revolutions.

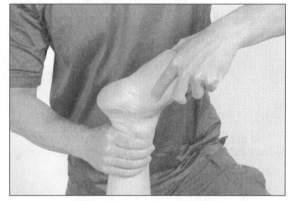

Holding her foot firmly, flex your partner's ankle.

Some receiver's ankles may pop and crack when you perform this range of motion, but if the rotations are not uncomfortable for your partner, continue, gradually loosening her ankle.

![Back Off]
Back Off

Do not massage feet where there is broken skin or a rash. You could push infection farther into your partner's system.

Another way of loosening your partner's ankle is done in the supine position; it is especially helpful in cases where your partner has worn high heels enough that her Achilles tendon at the back of her ankle has shortened:

1. Place your hand and lower forearm against the sole of her foot, cupping her heel in one of your hands.

2. Gently press her forefoot back toward her knee.

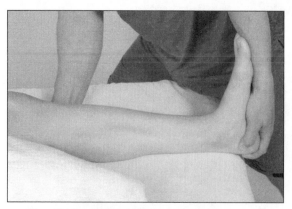

This ankle stretch is particularly good for women whose Achilles tendons have shortened from wearing high-heeled shoes.

3. Hold her foot in this position for about 10 seconds and then repeat the action 3 or 4 times.

Foot Massage Precautions

In addition to the Back Off sidebars in this chapter, here are a few other precautions to keep in mind when you're working on the feet.

Never use any kind of pointed pressure below the knees of a pregnant woman. Some acupressure points in her feet and lower legs have the potential of stimulating uterine contractions prior to the time she is ready to go into labor.

If your partner has numbness due to an illness like diabetes, don't use pointed pressure or deep techniques on her lower legs and feet. She might be unable to give you accurate feedback on how the pressure feels to her.

If you're massaging someone's lower legs and feet, and an area where you have exerted pointed pressure does not spring back quickly but retains an indentation, the person might have what is called *pitting edema*. This is a condition where there's a buildup of proteins and fluid in the tissues. Usually people don't have pitting edema unless they're suffering from a heart or circulatory problem. These problems can be serious, so a medical care provider should check the person.

The Least You Need to Know

◆ Massage is excellent for helping people with flat feet and plantar fasciitis.

◆ Massaging the feet can help relax tension in locations all over the body.

◆ You can help increase the range of movement of feet and ankles with massage.

◆ As wonderful as a foot massage can feel, keep some precautions in mind when you're dealing with the feet.

In This Chapter

- ◆ Easing leg pain and cramps

- ◆ Massage to help arm, hand, and chest pain

- ◆ Relieving aches and pains resulting from computer work

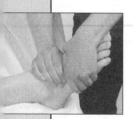 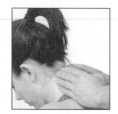 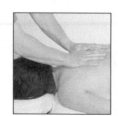 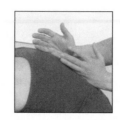 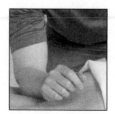 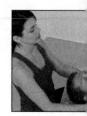

Chapter 17

Muscle Pains

Of all the benefits massage has for the body and its various systems, relieving muscular aches and pains is perhaps its best-known advantage. In this chapter, we give you ideas of how to use massage to help alleviate a variety of muscle-pain problems, from leg cramps to muscle aches from sitting at a computer all day.

Leg Cramps

Unfortunately, one of the most common and painful conditions that affects the legs—shin splints—responds only minimally to the increased circulation massage provides. Some other leg conditions that are uncomfortable, like varicose veins, prohibit the direct application of massage. (The techniques in Chapter 10 assist with tired and achy legs and thighs, and massage specifically for runners is covered in Chapter 18.)

Leg cramps often associated with pregnancy and "growing pains" in adolescence respond well to massage. If your partner is having immediate problems with calf cramps …

1. Apply pressure on the front of her foot by cupping the heel of her foot in one hand and using your forearm to flex the front of the foot toward her shin.
2. Apply pressure for about 30 to 45 seconds to release the cramp.
3. Perform petrissage on the calf to further relax the muscles so they don't cramp again. Start slowly and gently with the petrissage, as the muscles will be sore after the cramping.

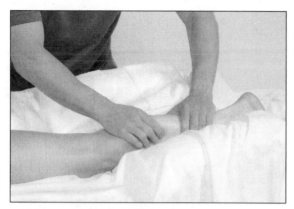

Apply petrissage to the calf to relax the muscles and help relieve leg cramps.

4. Gradually increase the depth and pressure, kneading and scooping the muscles from one of your hands to the other.

Sore Forearm and Hand Muscles

We use our arms and hands for almost everything we do, so it's not surprising that they get tired and sore from time to time. Discomfort in arms and hands comes from two sources: heavy lifting, pulling, or use of tools, which fatigue the arms and hands, and all the very fine movements associated with writing, keyboarding, hand crafts, and other repetitive tasks requiring dexterity. The discomfort is approached the same way, even though the cause of pain is different.

For general overuse, fatigue, and soreness of the wrists and forearms, follow the basic sequence for hands, arms, and shoulders in Chapter 8. After you've thoroughly warmed up your partner's arms and hands, begin to explore the muscles more deeply:

1. Use circular friction on the palm of her hand.

2. Using two fingers, begin to systematically and slowly apply relatively deep effleurage

strokes up her forearm. You won't cover much territory at a time with two fingers, but it will give you the opportunity to systematically search for knots, ropey bands, trigger points, and dense areas in the muscles on both sides of her forearm.

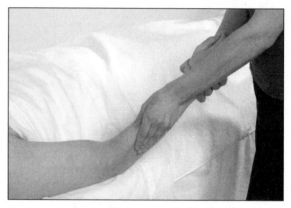

Applying effleurage to the forearm.

3. If you're making the strokes slowly enough, you'll be able to stop right where the focus of tension is; hold the area with moderate pressure for about 30 seconds, and ask her to breathe into the area you're pressing.

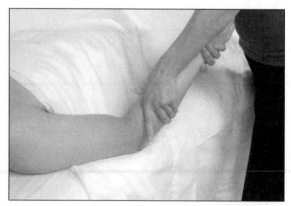

Applying petrissage to the forearm muscles.

When you really go searching for tight areas in the forearms, you're likely to find quite a few of them. Petrissage after the very specific work on tight muscles helps increase circulation and flush lactic acid from the tissues.

Carpal Tunnel

If your partner has some symptoms of carpal tunnel syndrome, such as a weakened grip and electrical-type shooting pains when the underside of the wrist is struck, you should probably seek clearance from her medical care provider before working on her wrist area.

When you've obtained clearance, you'll want to warm up the area with effleurage and petrissage. Then …

1. Open and close her hand, using one hand on the thumb side of her hand and your other hand on the pinky side to raise the edges of her hand up away from her palm and then squeeze her palm together.

2. Holding her hand so your thumbs are on the back of her wrist, apply firm circular friction there to loosen the retinaculum for about half a minute, a connective tissue structure that can hold the bones surrounding the carpal tunnel too close together, thereby compressing one of the nerves that serves the hand.

Office/Computer-Related Aches and Pains

Our bodies are designed for motion, and most of us, we authors included, sit too still for too long when we're in front of our computers. As a result, our bodies hold tension in certain sets of muscles that are held in contracted positions for extended time periods. The amount of tension depends, in part, on how ergonomically designed the workspace is. Most people who work at a computer hold their head slightly forward, with their necks held rigidly to see the screen. Frequently, their shoulders are elevated toward their ears. Shoulders may be rounded forward, and the computer user may sink into a

rounded lower back. All these positions result in tired and achy muscles.

The best solution, of course, would be to follow your hard day at the computer with a full-body massage. It goes without saying you may also want to evaluate your work station try to correct your posture at the computer, so you can have a massage purely for the enjoyment of it, rather than to relieve discomfort.

> **Press Here**
>
> Computers are probably one of the most significant contributors to the rise in the public's use of massage therapy and the rapid increase in the numbers of massage therapists working in the field (see Chapter 20).

Here are some specific techniques for a receiver who is experiencing discomfort from long hours at a computer. Working with your partner on a mat on the floor can allow you to exert downward pressure without putting strain on your own body. Some of these positions can be modified so that your partner is in a chair. How well that will work depends on the relative heights of the giver your partner, and the chair, but props like pillows or a footstool can help, if your partner is not flexible enough to sit comfortably on the floor.

1. Stand behind your partner, who should be seated on a mat on the floor with her legs crossed or straight out in front of her.

2. With the outside margin of one of your feet forward (that is, pigeon-toed), slide your foot forward and support your partner's back with your lower leg.

3. Your other leg should be far back to give you stability as you lean your palms on her shoulders, gradually leaning more heavily with your fingers pointed forward and then out over the sides of her shoulders.

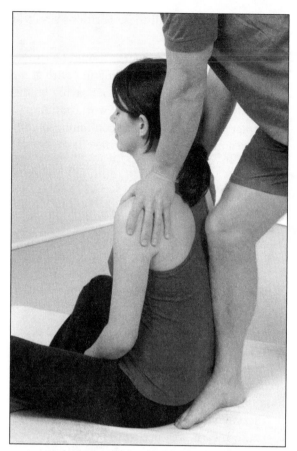

Press on her shoulders with your palms. Note the use of your leg to stabilize her back.

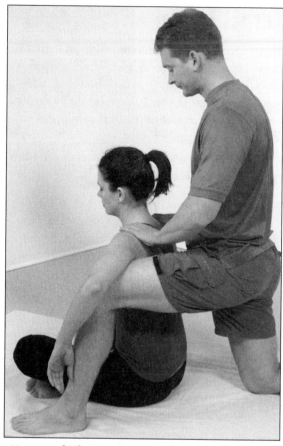

Use your thigh to support your partner's arm before working on her shoulder.

4. Palm her shoulders in this way about four times in each position.

5. Sink down on one knee, supporting her back as you do so.

6. Place your foot flat on the mat so you can put her left upper arm over your thigh. She should be comfortably upright.

7. Tilt her head to the left, and place your forearm where the right side of her neck changes angle at her shoulder, with your palm facing down.

8. Rotate your forearm to the right five or six times, starting each time at the same point at the base of her neck and rotating your arm so the palm of your hand goes from facing downward to facing upward.

9. Lean gently into the forearm at first, gradually sinking your weight into the stroke.

10. Reach down, grasp her right elbow, and bring her arm up, taking her wrist in your left hand and keeping her elbow in your right hand.

11. Rotate her arm six or eight times, keeping her wrist and elbow roughly at the same level and working the edge of her stretch as your rotate her upper arm back toward you.

12. Place her hand behind her neck, and with your left hand, gently pull her elbow in a bit closer to her head.

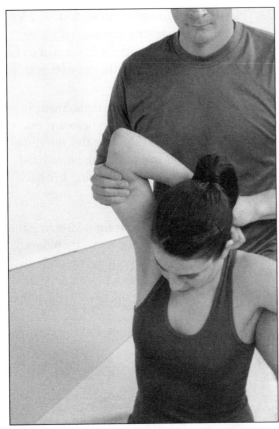

Lift your partner's elbow and place her hand behind her neck.

13. Using the entire palm of your hand to prevent pinching, squeeze the back of her arm up and down the triceps muscle.

14. Holding her elbow, place her arm back in her lap, and take her other arm off your thigh and place it in her lap.

15. Repeat on the other side.

16. Then slide down so you're kneeling with open knees behind your partner, supporting her shoulders with your hands as you change position.

17. Apply petrissage to her upper shoulder muscles, lifting and squeezing the upper trapezius muscles for a minute or two or until you feel a softening of the muscles.

18. Perform circular friction along the muscles to each side of her spine up and down her neck for about a minute.

19. Tilt your partner head forward and lace your fingers together, placing the heels of your hands on the sides of her neck and sliding them toward each other off the back of her neck.

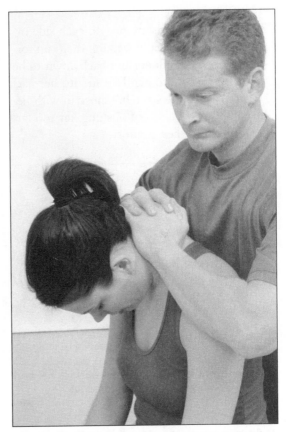

Use the heels of your hands to apply strokes to the back of your partner's neck.

20. Move up and down her neck, repeating this stroke in three or four more positions on her neck.

21. Apply petrissage to her deltoids, the muscles that cap the shoulders, squeezing the muscles and rotating her upper shoulders if they seem to be rigid.

22. Return to a kneeling position, lifting her arms over her head, and bring her into a forward bend.

23. Press both hands at once on each side of her spine, gradually walking them up to her upper shoulders and back down to her waist. Be sure to gently lean into her back to enhance the stretch. Check in with her to be sure you're not pushing her too far forward for her comfort.

24. Placing your forearms on each side of her spine, make a sawing motion with your arms up and down her back, parallel to her spine, creating heat in the muscles with the friction.

25. You may follow this with tapotement in the forward bend position before pressing her mid-back (not over the vertebrae!) with one hand and using the other hand on her upper shoulder to bring her back into an upright position.

This sequence is excellent for addressing the tension that builds up in the neck, shoulders, and upper back. Be cautious to not push her range of motion beyond her comfort level, and avoid rolling your arm on the bony areas of her upper shoulders.

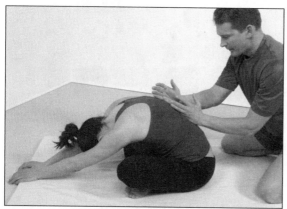

Bring her into a forward bend and work on her back with your hands and forearms.

The Least You Need to Know

◆ Many times, leg cramps can be relieved by using petrissage to relax the calf muscles.

◆ Massage can help with muscle pain in the arms, hands, and chest. It can even help some people with carpal tunnel problems.

◆ Long hours of computer work are bad for our bodies, but massage can help relieve the resulting pain.

◆ Massaging your partner on a mat on the floor can give you the benefit of being in a good position to exert downward pressure on her shoulders.

In This Chapter

- ◆ Easing stress and anxiety with massage
- ◆ Massaging away menstrual problems
- ◆ Using massage to treat common sports injuries
- ◆ Working on joint problems

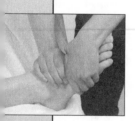
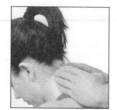
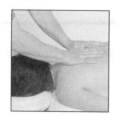
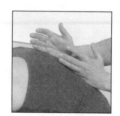
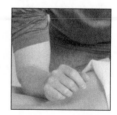
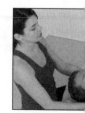

Chapter 18

General Conditions

In earlier chapters we talked about using massage to address specific problems, but massage is also useful in helping with what might be called whole-body problems, or in the case of stress and anxiety, body-mind conditions.

Massage is considered a holistic practice; that is, it addresses the whole person. We tend to think of our minds as separate from our bodies, but there is considerable connection at all levels. Massage can affect emotional and psychological states as much as it affects a person's physical body.

Stress and Anxiety

Your body responds to all kinds of stress in the same way, whether it's a car heading directly toward you at high speed or an important deadline at work. Your sympathetic nervous system is activated in what is commonly called the "fight-or-flight" response. This response provides for the bursts of intense energy needed when you must get out of the way of a speeding vehicle.

Meanwhile, numerous internal adjustments are designed to protect you from threats to your survival. Your blood leaves the core and rushes to your legs and arms to help you run fast or defend yourself strongly. Your pupils dilate and you become hypersensitive to all kinds of stimuli—visual, audible, and tactile. Your heartbeat becomes more rapid, and your blood pressure shoots up. Adrenaline and other stress hormones flood your body, and you're prepared for attack.

This is all well and good if you encounter a lurking saber-toothed tiger, but if the daily deadlines at the office, traffic, family crises, or conflict continually stimulate your sympathetic nervous system response, it may block the action of the other part of your autonomic nervous system function: the parasympathetic response.

Your parasympathetic nervous system, where your relaxation response is generated, is activated by periods of calm rest and nurturance. Energy is conserved and applied to your maintenance, renewal, and repair needs. Your heartbeat slows, digestion is supported, and your energy reserves are replenished. The two autonomic nervous system functions are complementary and they balance one another. You need extra blood in your legs to run fast, but if you're going to be the tiger's lunch, digesting your own might not be a high biological priority at the time.

Press Here

Nature has designed our body so perceived threats to our well-being take precedence over routine "maintenance" activities, like digestion.

Massage is precisely the type of relaxing activity that supports the renewal and repair functions of your body.

The alarm stage of the fight-or-flight response may be necessary on occasion. But if you don't have time to regroup from its effects, and if you don't get a break for true rest and renewal, exhaustion sets in during the resistance phase. Too much sympathetic nervous system activation can develop symptoms such as sweating, digestive difficulties, anxiety, trembling, dry mouth and throat, increased blood pressure, a pounding heart, and other uncomfortable conditions. And that's just in the short term. If long-term stress persists, your muscles become chronically tight. This constricts blood flow and oxygen delivery to your muscles, increasing pain, reducing strength, and fostering the development of trigger points. You may end up with high blood pressure, decreased immune responses, and, therefore, more illnesses, an altered metabolism, and more likelihood of headaches, thinning bones, ulcers, difficulty sleeping, and emotional sensitivity—just to name a few long-term consequences.

Back Off

While the short term effects of stress can be very uncomfortable, the long-term effects can be life-threatening. Stress contributes to the development of many diseases, and it worsens pain. Contributing to the relaxation response, massage can help prevent disease conditions, and may reduce existing pain.

Massaging Away Stress

Apply massage to a person who is experiencing any stage of the fight-or-flight response and you'll begin to activate calming and restorative effects from activating the parasympathetic nervous system. Your partner's breathing will slow. Her digestion will rev up, and you will likely hear her digestive tract noises as she begins to relax. Often there will be a discharge of energy in the form of her limbs jerking as she sinks down into relaxation at the edge of sleep. She will tend to visibly melt into the table or mat as you massage her.

It is important when massaging people who are in any stage of the stress response to be especially grounded and peaceful in your own center. You can't give what you don't have, so be sure to take time to get centered, focused, and grounded as we detailed in Chapter 3, and to pay attention to making your massage environment as serene and calming as possible, as discussed in Chapter 2. We are like tuning forks or bells; when a tone is struck on one, another near it will begin to vibrate with the same tone. If your intention is strong to help another person become calmer and you are in a serene frame of mind, your partner will experience at least a vacation from stress and anxiety for the time you're massaging her, and perhaps much longer. Sometimes all people need is an interruption in a dysfunctional "loop" to which they've become accustomed.

To begin relieving stress through massage, place three fingers across the bottom of your partner's breastbone (sternum). Then take one finger and press into the middle of the bone right above your highest finger. This point is an acupressure point called the Sea of Tranquility, named for its effect on a person. Hold this for about 30 seconds, encouraging your partner to breathe deeply and evenly.

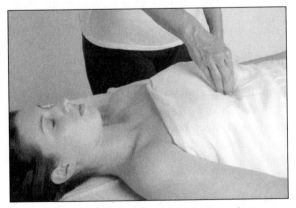

The Sea of Tranquility acupressure point.

Another useful acupressure point for stress and anxiety is the third-eye point, between your partner's eyebrows and slightly above the bridge of her nose.

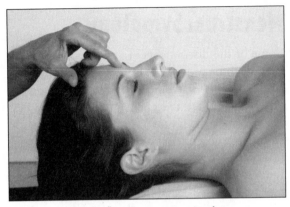

The third-eye acupressure point.

Press Here

We are like tuning forks for one another. If you are relaxed and at ease, the person you are massaging will tend to sink into a similar level of relaxation. Massage can help interrupt accustomed stress and let your partner feel there is another option to being keyed up all the time.

Check out the acupressure directions in Chapter 19 for specific information on how to apply these points.

Other than some acupressure points for stress and anxiety, no specific techniques target these conditions, but the way in which you implement massage for a stressed individual makes all the difference in how quickly and fully she responds. Encouraging her to breathe deeply and slowly into her abdomen is very helpful when combined with slow and nurturing massage strokes.

Menstrual Symptoms

Some of the discomforts of a woman's monthly cycles can be relieved by massage. In addition to the distraction from pain provided by gentle effleurage on her abdomen, a woman might benefit from the use of a heat pack in the area to ease her discomfort. There are acupressure points all over the sacrum that can assist in reducing abdominal pain as well as pain in her hips and lower back.

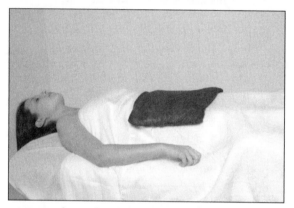

Heat packs on the abdomen can help relieve menstrual cramps.

Many women experience heightened irritability and more intense emotional reactions like anger and sadness right before and during the first few days of their menstrual periods. A comforting and calming massage can help calm a woman's emotional and physical being, so she's not so "on edge."

There seems to be a link between major hormone shifts and "touchiness" in some women, demonstrated by some women who become so edgy during their periods that the stimulation of being touched makes their tension and unsettled feelings more pronounced. This is also true of pregnant and laboring women and menopausal women who are experiencing hot flashes.

If you're massaging your partner at any time and she seems to become more tense during her massage, it's best to ask her directly if she wants you to continue or whether you need to change the way you're massaging her. Conditions other than hormonal ones can also trigger irritability and oversensitivity, including the actions of some prescription medications.

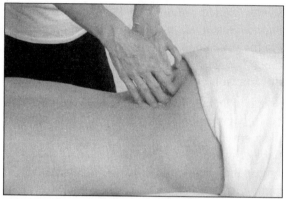

Pressing the sacral points can ease menstrual cramps, as well as lower back and hip pain.

A number of acupressure points can assist with menstrual discomforts, both physical and emotional. See Chapter 19 for acupressure technique.

Postworkout Massage

Evenly applied post-athletic massage aims at removing waste products from the muscles and involves no deep pressure. Apply light effleurage and petrissage strokes repeatedly to any area that's sore and fatigued from physical activity.

Back Off

Shin splints are a very common injury, and they may be associated with several different types of lower-leg injury, which you should not massage.

Gently stretch out a muscle that cramps due to athletic activity. This will be particularly common in the calf muscles, which we covered in Chapter 15.

When Massage and Sports Injuries Don't Mix

As great as a massage can be after a hard workout, if you massage an athlete with injuries you will need to take precautions to avoid making their conditions worse.

Do not perform any massage on minor sports injuries, such as strains or sprains, until at least 48 hours have passed. If the injury is debilitating, you should avoid applying massage techniques until a physician examines the athlete. Do not apply any strokes to an area where there is swelling. When the athlete is cleared by his physician to receive massage to the area of a strain, start with light effleurage strokes in the direction of the muscle fibers, and gradually deepen the strokes—but always stay within your partner's comfort level.

At Your Fingertips

Apply ice in a small circular pattern on any area of redness from a blow for up to a minute at a time. This helps keep a minor bruise from developing further. Otherwise, you should not massage a bruise.

When the injury is largely resolved but is still causing some stiffness or lingering discomfort, it will be fine for you to apply all the massage techniques we have discussed for that area. Among these, friction helps restore flexibility and pliability more than other strokes, but always use effleurage and petrissage to warm up the tissues before applying friction to the area. Then apply effleurage and petrissage again after friction.

Joint Issues

As the population ages, more and more people experience the kinds of impaired movement and discomfort that come from decades of joint wear and tear. *Arthritis* is a term that applies to about 100 conditions that affect people's joints. Only one, *osteoarthritis*, is caused purely by wear and tear. It is the most common form of arthritis, with about 20 million Americans suffering from it. Fortunately, unlike many of the other arthritic conditions, osteoarthritis does not create much inflammation or damage to other parts of the body and, therefore, you can safely massage a person with osteoarthritis.

Back Off

Massage techniques should not be applied to areas where a joint has been injured or hurt in a way that has resulted in inflammation. You can recognize inflammation by the presence of redness, swelling, heat, and pain. Massaging an inflamed area anywhere in someone's body has the possibility of damaging the tissues or spreading infection.

As long as you avoid massaging a joint that shows signs of redness and swelling, massage usually makes someone who has osteoarthritis feel better. This is in part due to the fact that people who are in pain tend to become tense, and this in turn makes the pain worse. When you can help your partner relax, you will, by that action alone, reduce their pain level.

In addition, when a person has pain in a joint, his muscles in the area of the joint tighten and sometimes go into spasm due to the joint pain. This becomes a cycle of pain, spasm, and more pain; you can use massage to interrupt this cycle by performing effleurage, petrissage, and friction in the affected area. Increased circulation to the area around an arthritic joint provides removal of irritating wastes produced by muscle spasm, and increases nutrition to the cells in the area and delivery of oxygen to the joint.

Back Off

Do not massage a joint that has been surgically replaced with an artificial joint, such as a knee or hip, until your partner has fully recovered from surgery and has been cleared for massage by her physician. You should not apply range-of-motion techniques to a limb that has an artificial joint.

Likewise, joint problems not related to age and wear and tear, like dislocations, require medical attention. Do not massage these areas.

The Least You Need to Know

◆ Massage is very effective in producing a relaxed state in which the body can rest and repair itself.

◆ The use of massage, heat, and acupressure points can relieve menstrual discomforts.

◆ Sports massage is generally not as deep as you would think, but uses superficial repetitive strokes to help muscles recover.

◆ Massage can decrease pain by increasing circulation in areas with arthritic joints.

In This Part

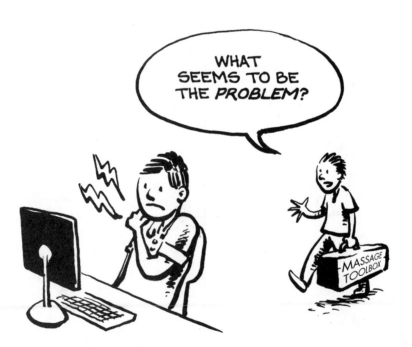

Taking It Further

In Part 4, we give you tips on enhancing the massage experience beyond the techniques and tools covered in the first three parts. While many of you won't be going into massage as a profession, we want to make that as easy as possible for those who choose this path. In the final chapters, we provide information for those who might want to make massage a full- or part-time career.

In This Chapter

- ◆ Running hot and cold
- ◆ Mixing water with massage
- ◆ Adding in acupressure
- ◆ Filling your massage toolbox

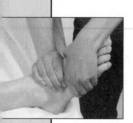
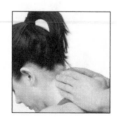
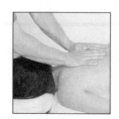
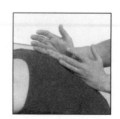
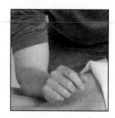
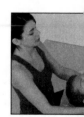

Chapter 19

Employing Enhancements

Many possible massage enhancements can add different dimensions to the overall massage experience. In this chapter, we take a look at the effects of heat, cold, water, and various tools. Heat, in particular, has a tremendous effect in promoting whole person and specific muscle relaxation. Heat can be applied in a number of ways, including with water. Water can be used as the carrier for relaxing warmth, and has the added benefit that it supports your partner. Heat not only makes a massage more relaxing for your partner; it loosens muscles enough to reduce the amount of pressure required of you to relax tight muscles.

Cold is used in cases where there is injury to tissues, or swelling, either in the case of injuries or in areas like the sinuses.

You're Getting Warm ...

Tight muscles and the connective tissue that surrounds them respond very well to heat. Effective applications of heat to the body begin to loosen tight muscles before you even begin to massage them. This can make the massage of a large-muscled or tight-muscled receiver much easier on your hands. The application of moist heat also increases your partner's comfort and relaxation level. A relaxed receiver is easier to massage.

To warm your partner's neck, place a pack under her neck when she's in the supine position. Hump up in the middle, if necessary, to support the curve of her neck.

Most commercially available heat packs are filled with small beads that suck moisture out of the air and release it slowly after they're heated in a microwave. Make your own packs by filling a large tube sock with uncooked rice and tying the end of the sock closed, or by filling different sizes of small pillowcases with rice and sewing them shut. The rice, like the filling in commercial packs, wicks moisture out of the air and provides moist heat.

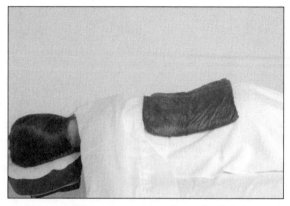

A heat pack on your partner's lower back helps with back pain.

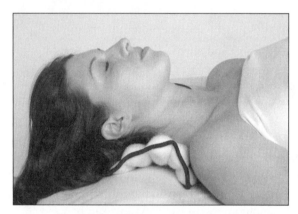

Use a heat pack under your receiver's neck to help loosen tight muscles prior to massage.

A large pack on the back helps loosen tight muscles up and down the side of her spine. You can place a pack on her back when she's in prone (face down) position. Or, if you're going to be working on her in the supine position place the heat packs on the table or mat and have your partner lie on them. Remove the heat pack from under her neck when you begin to massage her face and neck.

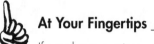

At Your Fingertips

If you have a microwave close by, reheat the pack while you're massaging her face and neck so you can reapply it after you've completed the massage there.

When using commercial heat packs, be sure to follow the manufacturer's directions. Some packs have a warning to not reheat them more than twice in one day. This seems to relate to the beads inside the packs not having enough moisture. In humid climates, there seems to be no limit to the number of times you may reheat a pack in a day.

Back Off

Beware of too-hot packs. Before placing a heated pack on your partner, check it by placing it on the underside of your forearm for at least 10 seconds. If it's too hot, place a towel between the pack and your partner. Be sure and ask your partner how the temperature of the pack feels to her; everyone has different levels of sensitivity to heat.

Cold has some utility, but it lacks the comforting and relaxing qualities of heat. At times, however, cold is useful, such as the brief application of cold to a recent injury site. A cool compress over your partner's eyes when her eyes are tired, red, and hot can be a great comfort, and the weight of the pack can help relax her eyes as well. Similarly, a cool compress helps some receivers' sinuses feel less sore. However, an equal number of people experience relief from a warm, moist compress. Try both and see which she prefers.

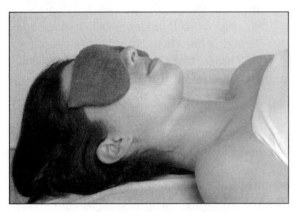

An eye pack can be very relaxing.

For vascular or migraine headaches, heat and cold can be combined for greater effect:

1. Place your partner's feet in a large dishpan or foot spa full of water as hot as she can tolerate comfortably.

2. Add very cool compresses on her forehead and the back of her neck.

At Your Fingertips _____

When you use ice on a painful area, do so for only a minute and keep the ice moving.

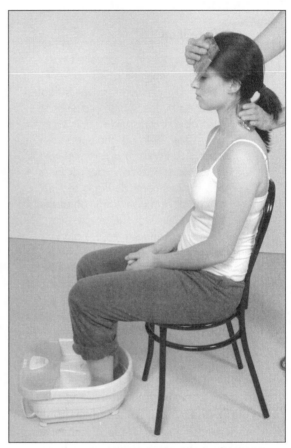

Use heat and cold at the same time to help with headaches.

Waterbreath Dance

Warm water is one of the most relaxing things we can apply to our bodies. Have you enjoyed a hot shower or a leisurely soak in the tub recently? Yes? Then you know what we mean.

If you have access to a hot tub and can adjust the temperature of the water, you can do some simple things that approximate some of the simpler moves of *Watsu*, a form of warm pool aquatic bodywork based on Zen *shiatsu*. The temperature of the pool should be in the range from 94° to 97°F.

Definition

Watsu is a form of aquatic body-work performed in a 94° to 96°F warm pool. The passive receiver is floated and stretched by the Watsu practitioner, who also applies pressure to points on the body. Being held up and supported in the water makes Watsu a very nurturing experience, in which flows from stillness to graceful movements during a session, which is usually an hour long. **Shiatsu** is a Japanese term for "finger pressure." It involves direct finger pressure along energy lines and specific points on the body to assist in the flow of life energy, called Qi. This energy flow supports body, mind, and spirit. Zen shiatsu adds the application of stretching the body along the energy lines.

1. Supporting your partner's neck securely with the curve of your elbow, and with your hand over the front of her shoulder on her deltoid muscle, place your other arm, with the palm down, under her hips.

2. Breathe with her as she breathes, and allow her body to sink with her exhalations, rising gently on its own with her inhalations.

3. Of course, don't allow her head to sink with the exhalations; you must watch her face to be sure her head is in the water over her ears, but not into her eyes, mouth, or nose. You'll experience moving up and down with her movements as her buoyancy changes with her breathing. You should match your breathing to the rhythm of her breath, if it is not too much of a strain for you.

4. After you've allowed the waterbreath dance, as it is called, to move her up and down for 6 to 10 cycles of breath, or until you feel her begin to noticeably relax, move her body toward her feet with an exhalation and then back to center on the inhalation.

5. On her next exhalation, repeat by moving her body in the direction her head is pointing. Gradually increase the back-and-forth motion in slow, small, gentle arcs up to the limits the tub allows. The movements will probably be several inches.

6. Experiment with gentle twists, or by putting your arm under one knee for some arcs and then under the other. Try placing one of your arms under her knees and bringing her knees closer to her chest a few times, being sure to support her neck in a neutral position, not flexed forward or allowed to hang back.

All movements should be very slow, fluid, and gentle, never pushing the limit of her range of motion in any direction. Support her neck and knees, and apply acupressure or simple compression on her neck, shoulders, and face. (See the following "Acupressure" section.) Be creative. This aquatic massage is purely for relaxation, and the amount of time you perform the movements or the number of times you apply compressions depends on how your partner responds to the experience.

Back Off

If your partner has any problems with motion sickness, move her very slowly, and concentrate more on pressure points. Be sure she knows she should alert you immediately if she begins to feel any nausea, or if anything is uncomfortable, particularly the angle of her neck. It's very easy to hyperextend a person's neck in the water or to allow her head to drop too far back, and you must constantly be vigilant to prevent this from happening.

At Your Fingertips

When doing any work in water, always have a thermometer to check the temperature. It should not exceed 97°F.

Acupressure

Acupressure was first developed 5,000 years ago in China and has been refined over the years. Needles, heated cones, or electrical impulses in traditional Chinese medicine and acupuncture stimulate the same energy pathways, called meridians, and particular points along the pathways. In acupressure, you can compress key energy points on the skin's surface with your fingers to stimulate your body's natural healing abilities. It can be used equally well on yourself or on others.

You can use different kinds of pressure on the points we detail here to achieve different results. Firm, prolonged pressure, from 1 to 3 minutes, is the most common type of acupressure application. You locate a point; sink in gradually with your finger, thumb, heel, or side of your hand; and hold it for at least 1 minute to calm and relax the nervous system. Interestingly, you apply pressure for only 5 seconds or so if you want to stimulate rather than relax a point or an area. Rapid tapping on a point is even more stimulating, and it may improve sluggish nerve and muscle function.

The depth to which you sink into a point should be enough to cause your partner to perceive it as a "good hurt"—a bit tender but so it feels as if it's doing some good. If you're focused and sensitive, you'll notice that different points have different feelings. Some feel as though they're soft, yielding points that draw you in; these points may be low energy points just "asking" for you to "top them off" with some energy. Other points feel hard, almost vibrating with excess energy.

Different bodies and different areas of one body require different amounts of pressure, so you'll want to concentrate on what you're doing and be sensitive. Heavily muscled individuals require deeper pressure than very thin or elderly individuals.

Press Here

If you seek to find a point that corresponds to a problem your receiver is having, it will likely feel tender or sore to your partner.

It's important that both you and your partner breathe fully and deeply during the application of acupressure. Your partner's deep breathing allows the points to release pain and tension and promote the flow of healing energy throughout the body. Your partner will feel her ability to regulate the steady amount of pressure you're exerting with your finger, as the pressure increases on her inhalations and decreases with her exhalations, regardless of where on the body you are pressing. Your deep and steady breath will not only help keep you focused and centered on what you're doing, but will also remind your partner to maintain a steady breathing pattern.

Now let's get hands-on with some acupressure points.

Sea of Vitality

These four points, two on each side of the spine, are right below the last rib (about ½ to 1 inch above the waist line), two finger widths and four finger widths away from the spine. These points are useful for relieving lower back pain.

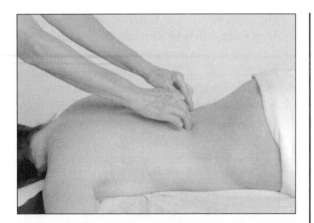

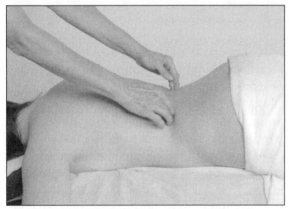

These four Sea of Vitality pressure points can be used to relieve lower back pain.

Third Eye

This point is in the indentation at the bridge of the nose between the eyebrows. This is a useful point for relieving anxiety, stress, chronic fatigue, and headaches. (See Chapter 18 for a photo.)

Gallbladder 2

This fingertip-size point where the top of the ear joins side of the face is useful for alleviating headache pain, especially vascular headaches and migraines.

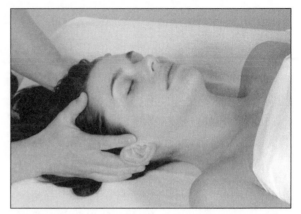

The Gallbladder 2 pressure point can be used to help with headache pain.

Heavenly Pillar

This pair of points is one finger width below the base of the skull on the prominent neck muscles about ½ inch out from the spine. These points are helpful for relieving stress, overexhaustion, insomnia, headaches, eyestrain, and stiff neck.

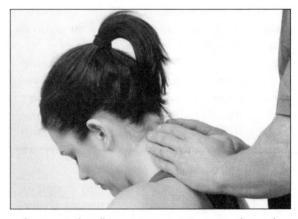

The Heavenly Pillar pressure points are on the neck.

Sea of Tranquility

This point is three finger widths from the bottom of the breastbone (sternum). It's helpful in the relief of tension in the chest, anxiety, nervousness, and depression. (See Chapter 18 for a photo.)

Shoulder Well

This point is on the highest part of the shoulder, slightly closer to the neck than midway between the base of the neck and the outer point of the shoulder. It relieves anxiety, fatigue, shoulder tension, and headaches.

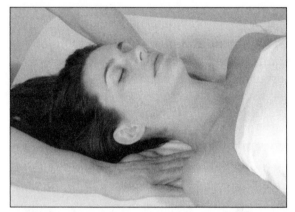

The Shoulder Well point is on top of the shoulder.

Letting Go

This point is about four finger widths up from the armpit crease and about one finger width inward on the outer part of the chest. It relieves congestion, coughing, shallow breathing, chest tension, and depression.

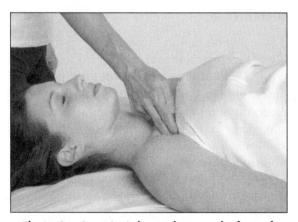

The Letting Go point is lower down on the front of the shoulder.

Supporting Mountain

At the bottom of the prominent calf muscle, about halfway between the knee crease and the heel, is where the Supporting Mountain point is located. If you glide your fingers up the back of the lower leg from the heel, your fingers will generally slow or stop right at this point.

It's useful for relieving calf cramping, foot swelling, and knee pain. In some individuals, it may also help relieve lower back pain.

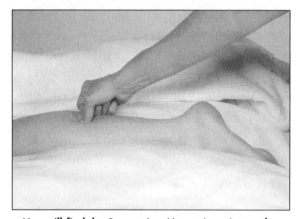

You will find the Supporting Mountain point on the back of the calf.

Sacral Points

These points are all over the sacrum in its indentations between the lower back and the tailbone. These points are useful for relief of menstrual cramps and frequently help lower back and hip pain as well.

Drilling Bamboo

These points are in the indentation of the inner eye socket just below the middle point of the eyebrows. They relieve sinus pain and congestion and eyestrain.

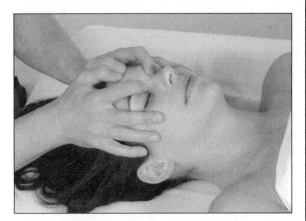

The drilling bamboo pressure points.

Welcoming Perfume

These points are just to the sides of the nostrils, by the nasal crease. These points are good for sinus congestion and pain.

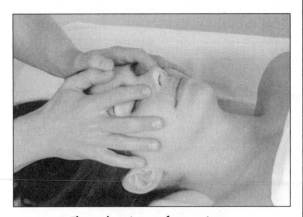

The welcoming perfume points.

Press Here _____

Your partner will probably need to breathe through her mouth when you apply pressure on the Welcome Perfume points, as it can close off the nostrils.

Facial Beauty

These points lie directly below the pupils of the eyes as your partner is looking straight ahead, just under the edge of the cheekbone. These points help sinus pain and congestion, as well as eye fatigue.

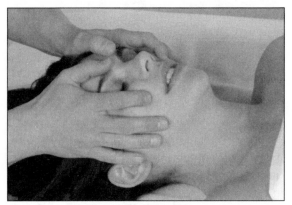

The facial beauty points.

Intermediary

These points are four finger widths up the middle of the underside of the arm from the wrist crease. They relieve and in some cases prevent upset stomach, nausea, and vomiting. They are especially good for preventing motion sickness, and you can even find elastic bands with little knobs to wear on your wrists when you're going to be in a situation that may cause you to have motion sickness.

Acupressure Precautions

Without professional training, never use abdominal points, as many disease conditions can exist for quite a while before your partner is aware of them, and your pressure could cause harm.

Avoid abdominal, lower-leg and foot, and middle-thigh pointed pressure in pregnant women.

Never apply any finger pressure in a jarring or abrupt way.

Avoid areas of broken skin or recent scars. You can apply pressure on points on the opposite side of the body, or opposite limb, which may have what is called a reflex effect, affecting both the side of the body you're working on and the same area on the other side of the body, due to the fact that both sides are served by the same set of nerves from the spinal cord.

And as with any massage, if you're not certain what you're dong won't cause any harm, don't do it.

Hand Tools

Some commonly available tools can assist those with less strength or stamina. Here are our favorite massage tools and some tips on how to use them.

Knobbles

The Knobble is a small, simple, rounded wooden tool you can use in the palm of your hand to exert pressure on areas that might need a bit more deep compression. Most tools for massage are useful for people whose fingers *hyperextend*, and Knobbles are no exception. Be cautious about the amount of pressure you use with a knobble or any other tool; you cannot feel with tools as you can with your fingers.

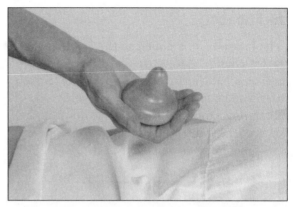

The Knobble is a simple but useful tool.

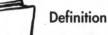

Definition

Hyperextension is when your fingers bow back toward your wrist rather than remaining in a straight line when you exert pressure with them.

In addition, Knobbles are very useful little tools to use on yourself. You can put one against the space between your scapula and your spine—a very common achy spot—and lean back in a chair with the Knobble between that spot and the back of the chair. Or you can place a Knobble on the floor and lie on it to apply pressure to any uncomfortable muscle in your back or hip area.

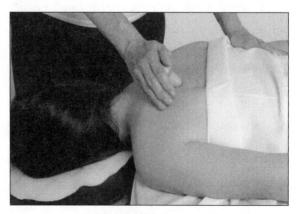

The Knobble in use.

Jacknobbers

The Jacknobber is similar to the Knobble in that it's designed to be used in your hand (or against a hard surface for self-massage). It has four wooden balls on a compact frame made of metal rods. You can use it to slide down both sides of the spine over clothing, or use one ball at a time for pressure points.

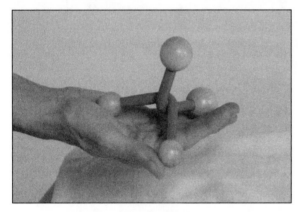

The Jacknobber.

The smaller two balls give a deeper effect for the same amount of pressure than the larger balls, and the tool is made so you can use it in a number of ways, picking those that work best for your hands. You can hold it with a thumb and forefinger exerting pressure on two of the balls, gripping the stems so you can press down with one ball, or even using two hands on the stems. Like the Knobble, it is a useful tool for self-massage, and particularly if you want to place it against a chair and stimulate pressure points on both sides of your spine at once.

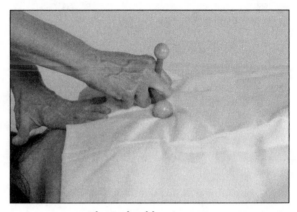

The Jacknobber in use.

Vibrating Massagers

Vibrating massagers really don't do very much for muscle discomfort and are frequently not very relaxing either, as they can provoke a tickle response or pull on body hair. Plus, the action they make is boringly repetitive, a They make an electrical noise that's not especially conducive to relaxation, and they have a techno edge that's not warm and nurturing like hands are.

The best we've found are percussion massagers, but they are only useful on broad areas like the back. Some vibrating massagers have an option to apply heat, and that's probably more useful than the vibration.

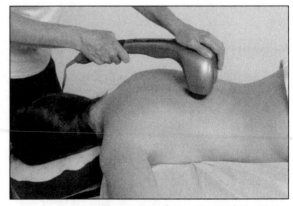

This percussive vibrator is only one type of electric vibrator.

Be careful about repeated use unless you have adequate hand protection. Prolonged or repeated use of these tools may lead to repetitive strain injuries like carpal tunnel syndrome.

Bongers

Bongers are fun toys. You place your thumbs and forefingers on the flexible shafts of these balls on sticks, and bounce the rubber balls up and down your partner's back, avoiding the kidney area. You can also use Bongers on your partner's calves, front and back thighs, and shoulders when your partner's in a seated position.

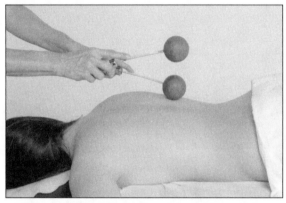

Think of playing a xylophone. That same action is what you do with Bongers.

Basically, Bongers are tools for performing tapotement if you can't seem to keep your wrists loose enough to avoid discomfort when using your hands. Like all the other tools, they can be good for self-massage, too. You can bong your own thighs, your upper shoulders, and your upper back pretty easily. Your arms simply aren't long enough to get to your upper back and shoulders, and Bongers effectively increase your reach.

Back Off _____

All tools should be used with the utmost sensitivity and excellent communication between you and your partner. Massage tools generally are hard, and you simply cannot have the sensitivity with a tool that you have with your fingers. When using tools, you must be extremely careful to avoid all bony areas, especially the spine.

The Least You Need to Know

◆ Heat and sometimes cold can be useful additions to your massage-technique inventory.

◆ Water massage can be useful in extending your repertoire of massage techniques.

◆ Learning the basics of acupressure can increase your massage skills.

◆ Inexpensive tools can help you save your hands and wrists and still provide a good massage.

In This Chapter

- ◆ Making massage a career
- ◆ Tips on learning to become a massage therapist
- ◆ Opportunities as a massage therapist
- ◆ Starting your own business

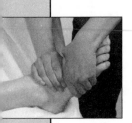
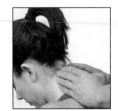
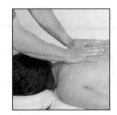
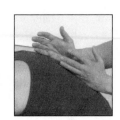
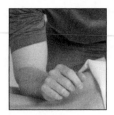
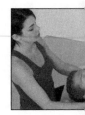

Chapter 20

The Next Level

If you read all the chapters in this book from cover to cover, and put the techniques shown on the book's DVD into practice, you will have some good massage techniques to share with friends or family members. For some of you, this might be as much as you want to do with massage.

But for others of you, this is just the tip of the iceberg. You want to learn more and perhaps make massage into a part-time or full-time career. Here are our thoughts and tips for you.

A Career in Massage

When asked about their massage experience prior to attending massage school, most students say they always massaged family or friends who enjoyed the experience. As they learned to give better massages, they have experienced how absolutely wonderful it is to help their loved ones with their aches, pains, and stress, and to access their inner healing resources. This is the route many of us have taken down the road toward a career in massage therapy. (What you've learned in this book in not massage therapy, but it provides enough information and guidance to allow you to give a satisfying and potentially health-promoting massage.)

However, it's a big step from casually helping friends and family to providing skilled touch in a professional manner for complete strangers. Massage therapy as a profession requires considerably more knowledge. You need to know more in-depth techniques, how to work with people who have pathological conditions (disease and dysfunction), human anatomy and physiology, and ethics. For this, you need hands-on instruction from professional instructors.

If you think massage therapy would be an interesting career, with potentially flexible hours, good pay, numerous options of work environments, and the opportunity to help others, you are absolutely correct. It is a career in which you can work in comfortable clothing (and often in bare feet!), have a personal meditative experience in each massage session, work in a serene and pleasant environment, have people appreciate you, get a good workout, and ... get paid for it.

Press Here

Few other fields, especially in health care, enable you to achieve your professional training and credentials in a year or less, for less than the cost of 1 year of higher education in-state at a college or university. It's a wonder everyone isn't stampeding to massage school!

The number of massage therapists in the United States jumped 27.9 percent from 2004 to 2006, from 188,527 practitioners to 241,058, according to Associated Bodywork and Massage Professionals (ABMP). The organization also reports that the massage industry generates $7 to $10 billion annually, and that consumers receive about 182 million sessions annually.

Does that mean there are too many massage therapists already? No. Demand for massage therapists is at an all-time high and is continuing to grow. The public's use of massage therapy as health care has tripled in the last decade. There are many reasons for this growth, such as the aging population of the United States, the public's changing view on health and wellness, and the state of the health care and health insurance system, to name a few. Massage therapy, along with allied health professions, has been identified as one of the top-growing professions in the United States in the next decade.

Becoming a Massage Therapist

Before you embark on a career as a massage therapist, ask yourself some serious questions:

- Do you like working with people?
- Do you enjoy caring for and helping others?
- Do you have, or are you willing to develop, strong communication skills?
- Can you comfortably work independently and remain quiet during most of your work?
- Are you willing and able to safeguard your own health and well-being by healthy exercise, diet, and sleep practices?

Your honest answers to these questions can help you decide if you should take the next step.

At Your Fingertips

Go get a massage! What better way to learn about the career than by getting a massage from one or more professional therapists? This gives you an opportunity to experience a typical massage session, and you can speak with someone who has personal knowledge of the field. (Many massage schools have student clinics where you can get a therapeutic massage without spending as much money as you would for a professional massage session.)

That next step could be taking a short introductory course. This will help you decide if massage school really is for you. While it won't provide you with enough training to qualify as a professional, such a course can give you a good idea of your commitment level and aptitude for the work. Typically running anywhere from a weekend to several weeks in length, introductory courses are offered through schools specializing in massage training as well as at community colleges, local YMCAs, hospitals, or other adult-education centers.

Schools, Licenses, and Tests

How much and what kind of training do you need? That depends on where you live and where you'll practice massage.

Look at the state laws in the area where you plan to practice massage therapy (see Appendix B). Thirty-four states require you to have a minimum of 500 hours of in-class education. Eleven states currently require more than 500 hours, and only 8 states do not formally regulate the profession. A few states, like California, lack state regulations but have areas within the state that regulate massage-therapy practice.

Most states, regardless of program length, require someone who has attended school for the number of required hours to take the National Certification Exam for Therapeutic Massage and Bodywork (NCETMB). Most states license massage therapists, and a few certify practitioners instead.

Press Here _____

If you're considering going into massage therapy in a state that currently doesn't regulate the practice, you must realize that 10 years ago, there was very little regulation of the field. Your chosen state will probably jump on the bandwagon of regulating massage before long. After all, it's a money making proposition for them to do so. And they are protecting the public by establishing standard credentials for those who perform massage therapy.

You have a variety of things to consider when choosing a massage school. Hopefully, any school in the state where you want to practice offers the number of course hours required by that state. Almost all schools are regulated by the state in which they are located. Ask if the schools you're looking at are state approved. Certain safeguards for your education are in place through state regulation.

Many career guides suggest you check on accreditation by a national accreditation agency. Such accreditation agencies include the Commission on Massage Training Accreditation (COMTA) and the Accrediting Commission of Career Schools and Colleges of Technology (ACCSCT).

But realize that these bodies accredit only 30 percent of all massage schools. The schools that can afford the high fees charged by the accreditation boards are frequently branches of huge conglomerate schools, and you might have a difficult time getting problems resolved at these schools because often the owners are elsewhere. Classes will tend to be large, as well. Community college programs are often less expensive than private massage schools, but classes are larger, and much of the coursework required is not as specific to massage.

Press Here _____

You might find that the small private school operated by owners who are not businesspeople per se, but, rather, are respected local massage practitioners, will have a better teacher/student ratio and may be more responsive to your individual needs.

You'll want to find a program that offers a well-rounded curriculum, with a balance between lecture and experiential courses. Look for a program that's very strong on the basics of massage and that teaches at least strong introductory material on various massage modalities in addition to a thorough grounding in basic Swedish massage and deep tissue massage. You'll need both a solid grounding in anatomy and physiology of the human body and ample opportunity to develop your touch skills. You also might want to consider a medical massage program, which has a focus on pathology, working with people who have diseases and disabilities.

Business and marketing courses are also important. It's fine to be knowledgeable about the human body talented and proficient in your hands-on work, but it's also essential that you develop interpersonal skills to help you identify and retain your clients, whether you're running your own business or working for someone else.

Another critical element of the school's curriculum should be student wellness training and an emphasis on the development of strength and good body mechanics, so you'll be able to practice your profession for many years to come. You might want to consider a school that includes yoga in its program of study.

Not only will a good school provide you with hours of hands-on training under the supervision of experienced massage therapists, but it should also offer you the chance to practice in simulated professional work situations. Well-designed schools usually operate a student clinic that accepts paying members of the general public as clients and/or maintain a comprehensive community outreach program where students can hone their skills.

At Your Fingertips

Get a couple massages at the student clinic of any school you're considering attending so you can find out what kind of therapists the school is producing. This also gives you an opportunity to talk with your student therapist about her experience and satisfaction with her school.

After Massage School Graduation

In our fast-paced, high-tech society, massage therapy can be a very rewarding choice if you're interested in helping people slow down, take stock, and improve the quality of their lives. As society becomes more and more mechanized, with electronic voices answering phones, online services, and even self-checkout at stores, an ever-increasing need for direct human contact is surfacing. Massage therapy is the ultimate high-touch, low-tech alternative for those who enjoy interacting with others on a uniquely focused personal basis.

After you've graduated from massage school, passed your national exam, and received your license or certificate to practice, your education is not over. You'll learn not only from the hours of practice in your profession, but also from the massage therapists you visit to maintain your own wellness.

Back Off

Massage is a physically demanding activity. Take care of yourself so you'll be able to take care of others longer and remain pain free. After all, if you believe in it for your clients, you'd better believe in it for your own well-being.

In most states, and to maintain national certification through NCBTMB, massage therapists are required to take 50 hours of approved continuing education classes over every 4-year period. This is no hardship, as the field of massage therapy is expanding and differentiating all the time, and many exciting and interesting continuing education classes are available. These classes boost your skills, keep your enthusiasm for your work high, and enhance your professional credentials. Sometimes your employer will even pay for your continuing education.

Working as a Professional Massage Therapist

As a professional massage therapist, you can be employed in a variety of settings:

- Massage therapy
- Alternative health care
- Pain or rehab clinics
- Chiropractor's, dentist's, and physician's offices
- Airports
- Health clubs
- Cruise ships
- Shopping malls
- Hotels
- Convention centers

And that's just the short list! You'll also find massage therapists working with professional sports teams, musicians and other entertainers, salons, resorts, and spas. Hospitals and nursing homes also employ massage therapists.

You'll have lots of employment opportunities if you decide to specialize. As research continues to prove the value of massage as a therapeutic tool, the variety and range of techniques and modalities you can learn expands. You might choose to focus on relaxation massage or take many hours of advanced training in clinical forms of massage. You might choose to work with a special segment of the population, becoming expert in the use of massage for infants, pregnant women, hospital patients, athletes, the elderly, or individuals in specific work situations. Some of your decisions will be dictated by your employment situation.

At Your Fingertips

To find a job, consult the school you attended, as area employers will often contact it, looking to hire graduates. The school should maintain a list of job opportunities. You can also search the local newspapers or go online to search for a job.

Starting Your Own Massage Business

If your dream is to be your own boss, a career in massage therapy can be the perfect way to achieve that goal. Keep in mind that being your own boss means you make *all* the decisions, from how many hours you work, how many clients you see, to how to set up your office.

Yes, this can be very liberating, especially if you have other commitments in your life, like a family, to consider. But you also have to make decisions on whether to incorporate your business, whether to do your own taxes or hire an accountant, and what fees to charge, and how you will get clients. You'll need to decide on location for your office, whether you want to share office space or employ other therapists, and a lot of other details. It can be very rewarding if you like business activities.

There's no doubt that the demand for massage is growing rapidly and the need for massage therapists will grow right along with it. If you have excellent massage skills, good business sense, and a dedication to service, you can expect to make a comfortable living.

Some massage therapists make as much as $100,000 per year, but the average income for a massage therapist is closer to $35,000. Part of this is because many massage therapists only work part time, or they work in spas or health clubs as a sub-contractor, giving part of their fees to the facility in which they work.

At Your Fingertips

If you want to work for yourself but hesitate to devote the time it takes to be a full-time massage therapist, consider doing it on a part-time basis. You can take satisfaction in helping others to deal with pain and stress while making some pretty good part-time income.

Starting a practice takes more time and effort than maintaining a thriving practice. You'll have to build up a fairly substantial client base, and that takes time. As in any business, it's usually the person who works the hardest and provides the best service who becomes successful. You'll need patience and perseverance to build a business from scratch, and you'll need to continue to develop the business skills you started learning in massage school.

Press Here

Massage therapy has a different standard from other types of work for what is considered to be full time: 18 hours per week of actual massage time. Of course, as a self-employed massage therapist, you'll have to be prepared to spend time managing financial records, filing taxes, doing lots of laundry, undertaking marketing efforts, and treating your massage therapy practice like the business enterprise it is. Generally, you'll spend anywhere from 30 to 50 minutes on other business activities for every hour you spend at the massage table. Of course, this changes over time.

If starting from scratch isn't appealing to you, consider jump-starting your massage business by making an investment in a massage franchise. You can also check into the possibility of buying an existing massage practice from someone who is retiring, leaving your area, or wants to sell his practice. Seriously consider consulting a lawyer and an accountant before undertaking either of these options, though.

When you have your own successful practice in place, regardless of the route you take to establish it, you might want to maximize your income opportunities by opening your own clinic or spa and employing other massage therapists.

More information is available through the major massage therapy organizations, Associate Bodywork and Massage Professionals (ABMP), and the American Massage Therapy Association (AMTA). In addition, remember the Small Business Administration, which provides free resources for new business owners.

While massage school training can be challenging, most schools are student-oriented and actively promote your learning. Having a private practice in massage therapy is a low overhead enterprise. Very few businesses require so little up-front expenses. Massage therapy is a very portable skill; people everywhere need it and want it. Because massage has received a lot of press in magazines, on the web, and by word of mouth in recent years, most people (your potential clients) know others who have had positive experiences receiving massage. And as you have learned, massage is a pleasant and rewarding activity to engage in, and it's always easier to work at something you really enjoy. Perhaps reading this book, watching the DVD, and practicing with your partner will inspire you to join the ranks of those of us who are dedicated to helping people, and are fulfilled in our work.

The Least You Need to Know

◆ Massage therapy is a great career if you get proper training.

◆ Most states are home to schools that offer massage therapy training.

◆ Starting your own massage business gives you control over your work schedule while making a comfortable income.

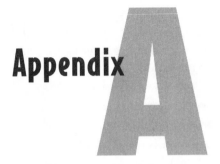

Appendix A

Resources for Supplies

Most communities today have one or more health food stores. Many of these stores also carry massage oils and creams, and some carry massage mats and other items. Many of the massage schools listed in Appendix B also sell massage supplies. If you can't find a local source for the items you need, you can certainly get them from one of the mail-order sources listed here.

www.comfortmassagemat.com
Ergonomic massage mat four-piece set pictured in book and video.

www.customcraftworks.com
Check here for massage tables, massage chairs, and almost any massage-related equipment and supplies you can think of.

www.bodyworkmall.com
A complete source for massage equipment and supplies.

www.massageking.com
Massage tables, massage chairs, and related items.

www.massagesupplies.com
All kinds of massage supplies.

www.massagewarehouse.com
A wide selection of items for massage, aromatherapy, chiropractic, etc.

www.earthlite.com
Handcrafted massage tables.

www.massageresource.com
Good, comprehensive resource directory for massage supplies and information.

www.herestherub.net
Massage tables, massage chairs, and related items.

www.biotone.com
Creams, lotions, aromatherapy supplies, etc.

www.kirlian.org/massage/livingearth/livindex.htm
Massage tables and accessories.

www.topmassagetables.com
Massage tables and accessories.

www.massageproducts.com
Massage tables and chairs, lubricants, aromatherapy, books, videos, etc.

www.source1medical.com
Massage tables, water therapy devices, etc.

www.sitincomfort.com
Massage tables, inversion tables, massage chairs, etc.

www.massagetherapy101.com
Massage therapy supplies and resources directory.

www.bodymindstore.com
Hot and cold packs, lubricants, tools, etc.

www.massageleader.com
Massage tables, massage chairs, and accessories.

www.massage-linen.com
Sheets for massage tables and related items.

www.mtso.ab.ca
Canadian source for massage tables and most other massage supplies.

Massage Schools

If you're interested in learning more about massage and possibly becoming professional massage therapists, you've come to the right place. This list of schools by state was accurate at the time of publication, but you may find additional listings at these search sites:

◆ Natural Healers (www.naturalhealers.com) and The Massage Resource (www.massageresource.com) are perhaps the most comprehensive listing of massage and other integrative healthcare schools.

◆ Dreaming Earth Botanicals (www.dreamingearth.com) is a nice source for aromatherapy products with a listing of quality massage schools.

Alabama

Red Mountain Institute
Birmingham
www.redmountaininstitute.com

Alaska

CB Healing Institute
Anchorage
www.cbhealinginstitute.com

Arizona

Arizona School of Integrative Studies
Clarkdale/Prescott
www.asismassage.com

Arizona School of Massage Therapy
Phoenix
www.arizonasmt.com

Desert Institute of the Healing Arts
Tucson
desert-institute.look4schools.com/1719-Tucson/
AZ.html

Phoenix Therapeutic Massage College
Flagstaff
www.ptmcaz.com

Rainstar University Therapeutic Massage Program
Scottsdale
www.rainstaruniversity.com/ctm.htm

Sedona School of Massage
Sedona
www.sedona-school-of-massage.com

Southwest Institute of Healing Arts
Tempe
www.swiha.com/tour.html

Arkansas

White River School of Massage
Fayetteville
www.wrsm.com

California

Academy of Natural Healing
San Clemente
1-800-399-3110, ext. 4252

Ahern's Massage Therapy School
Ahwahnee
www.ahernmassageschool.com

Arcata School of Massage
Arcata
www.arcatamassage.com

Ashland Institute of Massage
Ashland
www.aimashland.com

Body Mind College
San Diego
www.bodymindcollege.com

Body Therapy Center
Palo Alto
www.bodymindspirit.net/massage/therapists.html

Diamond Light School of Massage and Healing Arts
San Anselmo
www.diamondlight.net/home.html

Hands on Healing Institute
Tujunga
www.gotohhi.org/contact.html

Heartwood Institute
Garberville
www.heartwoodinstitute.com

Institute of Professional Practical Therapy
Los Angeles/North Hollywood
www.ippt.com

International Professional School of Bodywork (IPSB)
San Diego
www.ipsb.edu

Mendocino School of Holistic Massage and Advanced Healing Arts
Redwood Valley
www.mendomassageschool.com/contact.htm

Mueller College of Holistic Studies
San Diego
www.mueller.edu

Napa Valley School of Massage
Napa
www.napamassageschool.com

National Holistic Institute
Emeryville
www.nhi.edu

Phillips School of Massage
Nevada City
www.handsinharmony.com/PSM_Top1.htm

World School of Massage and Holistic Healing Arts
Pleasanton
www.worldschoolmassage.com

Colorado

Colorado Institute of Massage Therapy
Colorado Springs
www.coimt.com

Colorado School of Healing Arts
Denver
www.csha.net/index.html

Cortiva Institute
Broomfield
www.cortiva.com/locations/denver

Denver School of Massage Therapy
Aurora
www.denversmt.com

Golden Institute of Massage School
Golden
www.goldeninstituteofmassage.com

Heritage School
Denver
www.heritage-education.com

MountainHeart School of Bodywork
Crested Butte
www.visitcrestedbutte.com/businesspage.cfm?businessid=268

Rocky Mountain Institute of Healing Arts
Durango
www.instituteofhealingarts.com

Connecticut

Central Mass School of Massage and Therapy
Spencer
www.centralmassschool.com

Connecticut Center for Massage Therapy
Groton
www.ccmt.com

Muscular Therapy Institute
Cambridge
www.mtiweb.edu

Delaware

Deep Muscle Therapy School
Wilmington
www.dmtsmassage.com

Florida

Academy of Healing Arts
Palm Beach, Lake Worth
561-965-5550

American Institute of Massage Therapy
Fort Lauderdale, Pompano Beach
www.aimt.com

Educating Hands School of Massage
Miami
www.educatinghands.com/home.html

Florida Academy of Massage and Skin Care
Fort Myers
239-489-2282
www.famsc.com

Florida College of Natural Health
Orlando, Maitland, Miami, Pompano Beach, Sarasota
www.fcnh.com

Humanities Center Institute of Allied Health School of Massage
Pinellas Park
www.allalliedhealthschools.com/schools/ID3669

Sarasota School of Massage Therapy
Sarasota
www.sarasotamassageschool.com

Suncoast II Tampa Bay School of Massage Therapy
Tampa
www.suncoastii.com

Georgia

Academy of Somatic Healing Arts
Atlanta
www.ashamassage.com

Atlanta School of Massage
Atlanta
www.atlantaschoolofmassage.com

Rising Spirit Institute of Natural Health
Atlanta
www.risingspiritinstitute.com

Hawaii

Hawaii Healing Arts College
Kailua
verizonsupersite.com/hhacdirectcom/enter

Maui School of Therapeutic Massage
Makawao
www.massagemaui.com

Idaho

Moscow School of Massage
Moscow
www.moscowschoolofmassage.com

Illinois

**Alive and Wellness, Inc.,
School of Massage Therapy**
Moline
www.alivewellness.com/home.html

**New School for Massage, Bodywork, and
Healing**
Chicago
www.newschoolmassage.com

**Northern Prairie School of Therapeutic
Massage and Bodywork**
Sycamore
www.northernprairieschool.com

**The Soma Institute/National School of
Clinical Massage Therapy**
Chicago
www.thesomainstitute.com

Wellness and Massage Training Institute
Woodridge
www.wmti.com

Indiana

Alexandria School of Scientific Therapeutics
Alexandria
www.assti.com

Iowa

Eastwind School of Holistic Healing
Iowa City
www.eastwindschool.com

Kansas

Massage Therapy Training Institute
Kansas City, MO
www.mtti.net/

Kentucky

Lexington Healing Arts Academy
Lexington
www.lexingtonhealingarts.com

Louisville School of Massage
Louisville
www.stillpointinc.net

Natural Health Institute of Bowling Green
Bowling Green
www.natural-health-inst.com

Maine

New Hampshire Institute for Therapeutic Arts
Bridgton
www.nhita.com

Maryland

Baltimore School of Massage
Linthicum
www.universities.com/On-Campus/www.
Baltimore_School_Of_Massage.html

Massachusetts

Acupressure Therapy Institute
Quincy
www.acupressuretherapy.com

Bancroft School of Massage Therapy
Worcester
www.bancroftsmt.com

Central Mass School of Massage and Therapy
Spencer
www.centralmassschool.com

Massage Institute of New England
Somerville
www.mine-massageinstitute.com

Palmer Institute of Massage and Bodywork
Salem
www.palmerinstitute.com

Solidago School of Massage and Holistic Health
Amesbury
www.solidagoschool.com

Michigan

Irene's Myomassology Institute
Southfield
www.imieducation.com

Minnesota

CenterPoint Massage and Shiatsu Therapy School and Clinic
Minneapolis
www.CenterPointMN.com

Minneapolis School of Massage and Bodywork
Minneapolis
www.mplsschoolofmassage.org

Northwestern Health Sciences University Massage Program
Bloomington
www.nwhealth.edu

Missouri

Massage Therapy Training Institute
Kansas City
www.mtti.net

Nebraska

Omaha School of Massage Therapy
Omaha
www.osmt.com

Nevada

Nevada School of Massage Therapy
Las Vegas
www.nevadasmt.com

New Jersey

Academy of Massage Therapy
Englewood
www.academyofmassage.com

Academy of Therapeutic Massage and Healing Arts
Vineland
sjacademy2heal.com

Atlantic County Healing Arts Institute
Atlantic City Area
www.achaimassage.com

Healing Hands Institute for Massage Therapy
Westwood
www.healinghandsinstitute.com/abouthhi.htm

Health Choices Holistic Massage School
Hillsborough
www.health-choices.com/index.htm

Helma Institute of Massage Therapy
Saddle Brook
www.helma.com

Therapeutic Massage Training Center
Westfield
massagetrainingcenter.com

New Mexico

New Mexico Academy of Healing Arts
Santa Fe
www.nmhealingarts.org

New Mexico School of Natural Therapeutics
Albuquerque
www.nmsnt.org

Scherer Institute of Natural Healing
Santa Fe
www.schererinstitute.org

New York

Hudson Valley School of Massage Therapy
Highland
www.hvsmassagetherapy.com

Swedish Institute
New York
www.swedishinstitute.org

North Carolina

Body Therapy Institute
Siler City
www.massage.net/index.html

Center for Massage and Natural Health
Asheville
www.centerformassage.com/education/
massage_school.htm

Edmund Morgan School of Neuromuscular and Massage Therapy
Cornelius
www.edmundmorganschool.com

Ohio

American Institute of Alternative Medicine—Massage Therapy
Columbus
www.aiam.edu/03_massage.html

Oregon

Ashland Institute of Massage
Ashland
www.aimashland.com

Oregon School of Massage
Portland/Salem
www.oregonschoolofmassage.com

Pennsylvania

Baltimore School of Massage
York
www.bsom.com

National Academy of Massage Therapy & Healing Sciences
Kulpsville
www.nationalmassage.com

Pittsburgh School of Massage Therapy
Pittsburgh
www.pghschmass.com

Tennessee

Natural Health Institute
Nashville
www.natural-health-inst.com/index-nashville.
php

Texas

Phoenix School of Holistic Health
Houston
www.themassageschool.com

Virginia

Blue Ridge School of Massage and Yoga
Blacksburg
www.blueridgemassage.org

Washington

Bellevue Massage School
Bellevue
www.bellevuemassageschool.com

Brian Utting School of Massage
Seattle
www.busm.edu

Northwest School of Massage
Federal Way
www.nwsm.net

West Virginia

Mountain State School of Massage
Charleston
www.mtnstmassage.com

Wisconsin

St. Croix Center for the Healing Arts
Hudson
www.sccha.com

TIBIA Massage School
Madison
www.capw.org/tibia

Index